Advance Praise

I have worked hard to heal past traumas with the help of Atul Mehra. Through his vast knowledge and deep concern for his fellow humans, he has created yet another book that can change your life. This book shows us that every disease and negative thought contributes to achieving oneness and complete acceptance of self. Strange as that may seem, Atul beautifully describes the hidden secrets of the unconscious mind and its correlation between health and disease. The Need for Disease is a pathway to self-understanding and inner connectedness - a beautiful and compassionate book.

Denise Cassino,

Award-winning Author and Publisher

When physical or mental health creates difficulties, we feel unworthy. We are worthy of self-discovery, personal growth, and boundless love. With over 22 years of professional experience and research, Atul Mehra brings awareness to hidden patterns controlling our everyday life. The Need for Disease is a journey from unconsciousness to consciousness, disease to health and division to the whole. A truly inspiring and motivational book.

Carol Moxam,

Lifestyle Leadership Expert &

Author of "Life is a Special Event."

There has never been a more critical moment in human history to understand the need for disease than now. With the recent pandemic, more needs to be done to understand better how diseases develop, what they ultimately mean to our longevity and how we can naturally adapt to negating the ill effects.

The Need for Disease is a thorough examination of how we create our diseases while delving deep into the unconscious origins to discover paths forward to health restoration and the ultimate wellbeing necessary to live to our full potential.

The Need for Disease provides a unique theory that disease evolution begins at the sperm consciousness stage. This revolutionary thought process promises to open new pathways of thinking that can potentially change how medical professionals approach disease treatment and how we as a population can overcome long-term detrimental effects.

Written by noted psychotherapist Atul Kumar Mehra, this book examines how everything starts in the womb, allowing us to understand better the foundations of disease and how best to treat them.

Dr. William Rodriguez G.
Clinical Psychologist - Ecuador
Hypnotherapist GTH – Germany
Homeopath UNAG - Mexico

THE NEED FOR DISEASE

If you create your disease,
you can heal it too

by
Atul K. Mehra

The Need for Disease
Atul K. Mehra
Mehra Publishing
All rights reserved
First Edition March 2023
Copyright © 2023 Atul K. Mehra
Cover design © 2023 by David Arias

Requests for permission should be addressed to

atul@atulmehra.com

Paperback ISBN: 978-1-7772753-4-1
eBook ISBN: 978-1-7772753-5-8

This book is dedicated

To the loving memory of my father, Raghu Nath Mehra and also to my mother, Darshi Mehra.

About the Author

Atul Kumar Mehra is an author, international speaker and Registered Psychotherapist in Ontario, Canada. He is the director of the Jaagran Psychoanalysis and Wellness Center in Mississauga, Ontario, a Registered Professional Counsellor, and a member of the Canadian Professional Counsellors' Association (CPCA). He is also a member of the Canadian Association of Psychodynamic Therapy (CAPT), a member of the National Guild of Hypnotists (USA) and a member of the College of Registered Psychotherapists of Ontario, Canada (CRPO).

He has worked with thousands of clients with mental health issues for more than 20 years and has completed more than 25,000 sessions from simple Anxiety to Psychosis and everything in between. He has around a 90% success rate, including the disintegration of a tumour.

Additionally, Atul is a Naturopath, a member and founder of Esculapio alternative medicine school in Quito, Ecuador, and a qualified instructor of Autogenous Training of Self Hypnosis certified by Sociedad Ecuatoriana de Hipnosis terapeutica y Hipnopedia. He has been initiated as a Grand Master Reiki and Master Karuna Reiki.

Currently, he works with Colour Therapy and Holistic Healing and has extensive knowledge in Swedish and Thai therapeutic massages, Aromatherapy and Manual

Lymphatic Drainage, among other techniques. He has participated in many courses and workshops on Hypnosis, Hypnoanesthesia and NLP (Neuro-Linguistic Programming). His field of investigation is the human mind and how it works on subliminal messages with binaural tones and Inspirational movies to improve the quality of life. He has created a course on advanced Hypnosis techniques based on covert communication. He is creating a pathway to guide others through "yoga beyond duality."

Atul has participated in moderated panel discussion videos with Dr. John Gray (The author of Men Are from Mars, Women Are from Venus) on diverse topics and has spoken on the same platform as Dr. Deepak Chopra. He has written many articles in local magazines and newspapers such as Raiz, Salud y Vida and Familia. He has also appeared as a guest speaker on hundreds of TV and radio shows in different languages and as a keynote speaker for national and international conferences. Among his significant achievements are his studies in Analytical Hypnotherapy (Integrative therapy of depth psychology under Hypnosis and in Hypnosis) from Meersburg, Germany.

Since early childhood, Atul's dream has always been to connect with the Source; a dream finally realized when he accessed and experienced the deepest human conscious form as sperm consciousness. With over 20 years of experience working with the unconscious mind, Atul has gained deep insights into it and writes and speaks internationally on "The Need for Disease." Those experiences made him realize the importance of totality and further opened pathways to understanding the importance of pain and love as consciousness and not as emotions. He thus discovered the true purpose of life that has guided him to work with clients suffering from mental and physical ailments.

Atul was born in New Delhi, India. He obtained a master's degree from Delhi University. He now resides in Mississauga, Ontario, Canada, with his wife and two daughters. Atul has always had a love of writing and has published articles in several countries and several languages. He has published his book The Unseen Wisdom of the Unborn (Amazon best-selling Author) and is working on two other books – Addiction is Survival, Not Guilt and My Unconscious Self.

In his leisure time, Atul enjoys playing chess, reading, and writing. He also teaches yoga and dancing meditation and is a huge soccer fan. He loves to travel and meet people and is fluent in Spanish, English, Hindi, and Punjabi. He also speaks a little French. In the future, Atul hopes to continue authoring books, share his knowledge with a broad cross-section of people, and enjoy the love and company of his family.

Contents

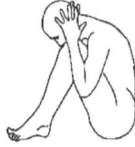

Acknowledgements

One of the essential things in life is to be grateful. We are all surrounded by so many blessings that we often ignore them completely. When we take awareness, we feel utterly fortunate to have those moments, experiences, things, or persons in our lives. Being grateful, showing gratitude, or acknowledgment is the symbol of happiness, satisfaction, and a good life.

The most prominent acknowledgment in my life is my parents, my father, Late Mr. Raghu Nath Mehra, who was my first teacher when I started developing analytical intelligence. I might be far behind where I am today without his teaching. Nevertheless, my very first gratitude in my life is to my mother, Mrs. Darshi Mehra, who nurtured me in so many ways, consciously and unconsciously, and without her, I would not be here today. The best moments of my life were when I relived and confirmed her unconditional love for me in her womb during my whole life therapy process. I am so blessed to have them both in my life, and if I ever retake birth, then without any doubt, they will be my first choice to select them as parents.

Life is more joyful and accepting if your family members support you. I have been so lucky to have my wife, Tatiana

Mehra, who sacrificed, loved me unconditionally, and helped me in good and bad times. My continuous source of inspiration is my two daughters, Anisha Mehra, and Ambar Mehra, who inspire me to share this knowledge because one day, I know this will help them find answers in their lives, although I will not be there.

Siblings play a significant role in life, and a good and trustworthy relationship with them provides us more fulfillment as we share everything with them from the womb. They are the proof and confidence of lifelong relationships. My gratitude extends to my siblings, Abhinav, and Rinku. They have always encouraged and supported me in all circumstances, with an extraordinary mention to my sister-in-law Pooja, my niece Anchal and my nephew Ariv.

Conveying the correct message in the book makes it worthy of understanding on much deeper levels, and it makes me so proud to have the unconditional support of Anjana Thom. She has helped me edit my second book with so much deep knowledge of the topic.

Friends are part of life, increasing the sense of belonging and purpose. Fortunately, all my friends are like an extended family to me. I am so grateful to know Kristy Higgins in my life, who has always been there in need, and her ingenuity and advice have helped me many times. My gratitude extends to Carol Moxam, who has constantly motivated and uplifted me to finish this book when I felt passionate procrastination and loyal laziness LOL.

Teachers are a constant source of knowledge, and they are guides in our life's journey. I want to extend my sincere gratitude to my teachers and friends, Dr. Jose Villalba and Late Dr. Werner Meinhold. Their therapeutic process helped me recognize and connect myself on the deepest level and the reconfirmation of self with many options.

My heartfelt and most profound gratitude also goes to my wonderfully creative and generous brother-in-law, David Arias, who diligently, once again, donated his time and expertise in creating a beautiful cover for my book.

I am also grateful to all those who have helped me write this book directly or indirectly, especially all my clients whose experiences during sessions taught me and motivated me to write this book. A special thanks to Denise Cassino of BestsellerServices.com.

Above all, I am eternally grateful to God, who has made it possible to write this book under his benign smile and divine guidance.

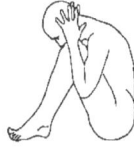

Foreword

As a clinical psychologist specializing in psychotherapy and differential diagnostics, I have seen many different forms of atypical disease presentation around the world. During my time at Princeton, I always wondered about the deeper and unconscious patterns that were revealed during some of my sessions. These patterns seemed to carry so much weight and energy - it was clear to me that they must have a fundamental impact on physical health as well.

I met Atul during my clinical project for the maritime industry. I had been writing new systems for intervention and treatment for seafarers, and Atul was one of the clinicians I consulted for cultural psychology. I was immediately impressed by his honest, calm, and authentic approach to the subject matter. He seemed well-adjusted and collected. I noticed rather quickly that he had worked a lot on himself to achieve this level of insight and openness. This person had taken a deep dive into his own past trauma and had somehow made darkness into light. We talked a lot about his own path of analysis and his insights. It was an honor to be given the luxury to ask questions about the important and difficult things in his life.

Therefore, it is with great pleasure and humility that I write about this book. The mind and body are one system and they always have been. It was practical, but a costly mistake to have separated body and mind during medical and psychological practices in the past. Atul is able to describe how early misguided relationships can set us up to a path of maladjusted emotional responses in the future that can have a huge impact on our physical wellbeing.

Our thoughts guide our response to stress and how we deal with it. Today's research confirms that people who think differently about stress have a different cardiovascular response to stress. It all starts and ends with how we think about things or how we have learned to think about things. This is just one more reason why this book is so critical during these times. Unfortunately, being well adjusted in our society hasn't been the best predictor for health. The reasons are explained by Atul very meticulously, and he is able to highlight how vital a holistic approach to health needs to be.

Self-love, Self-acceptance, and self-discovery can improve our health and lead to happier feeling and a better understanding of our origin. Love always needs to lead the way. This book is a true gemstone, and we need more books that help us go deeper into the meaning of the unconscious truth. I applaud all your hard work that went into writing this book.

Dr. Charles Watkins
Hamburg, Germany
Friday, August 12, 2022

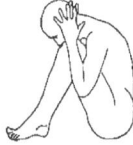

Foreword 2

I am deeply honoured to write this foreword for Atul Kumar Mehra and his latest publication, "The Need for Disease." This book allows the reader to take a reflective pause on aspects of their lives that provide a gateway into their healing process.

Atul's writing shares a perspective of the mental patterns that may create "dis-ease" in the body. It can be challenging to explain or understand the mental, emotional, and physical shifts that can take place throughout a therapeutic process that restores health and well-being. The following pages allow the reader to reflect on parts of themselves through stories and case studies to make the unconscious conscious and actuate the healing process.

I met Atul as the National Vice President of the Canadian Professional Counsellors Association (CPCA) in 2010. I recognized Atul's depth of knowledge, professional experience and ongoing growth and development in psychotherapy. Far too often, trained professionals from other countries do not receive the recognition they deserve. I supported his application to become a registered counsellor in Canada and was pleased to see him become registered under the Health Care Act of Ontario as a Registered Psychotherapist. As our professional relationship grew, so did my knowledge and understanding of integrative depth psychology concepts, learning more about unconscious resistance and deepening my understanding of psychodynamic therapy. This led me on a journey to Greece with Atul, where we spent an intensive week of training under the guidance of Dr. Werner Meinhold, learning about the therapeutic possibilities of hypnosis and its combination with depth psychology. As a published author, international speaker and practising psychotherapist, Atul shares this vital topic – the Need for Disease.

Understanding the psychological underpinnings of the Need for Disease can be essential to our healing and recovery. Atul's research and work brings different perspectives and concepts that enrich present day methods and therapeutic techniques. As the reader, I encourage you to be open-minded and take in the information that fits you. Atul's work challenges some of our patterns of thinking and opens the door to looking at our lives in a new way. As you read the Need for Disease, you will understand Atul's passion for uncovering the emotional and mental roots of our conditions. I encourage you to be curious, consider aspects of your Self, deepen your understanding, and connect to your higher wisdom for your own healing and recovery. "If we can create it, we can change it."

Kristy Higgins, RTC, MTC, RCS Registered Therapeutic Counsellor, Master Therapeutic Counsellor, Registered Counselling Supervisor -ACCT

*"Solutions were created before problems,
and problems are bridges to solutions."*

Atul Mehra

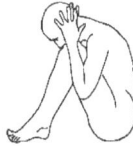

Preface

When I was four years old, my father taught me how to meditate and during that time, I had loads of questions that had disturbed the tranquillity of my life for so many years.

"Who am I?"

"What is the purpose of my life?"

"What am I doing here?"

"Why do I take birth and have to die one day, although I do not want to?"

"What is happiness, and what is sadness? Why does everybody want to be happy and not sad? What will happen if I try to be sad when I am happy and vice-versa?"

Can you imagine I had all these questions even before I turned ten years old? All those questions about my existence, relationships, health, and whatever else entered my mind. I remember waking up and wondering, "why it is, what is?"

I could not sleep for hours, and it began creating health problems as well as trouble for me in school.

I questioned everything: God, soul, body, mind and whatever else related. I remember those thought processes became so dominant that I lost my mental peace and began behaving in some bizarre way. I remember staring off into the emptiness but deeply absorbed into my thinking world. It created great mental exhaustion and wasted energy because I started losing interest in life and everything surrounding me.

Fortunately, my father was not only my first Guru but also a great friend and someone straightforward to talk to. I remember explaining my frustration and desperation to get answers that night. He listened to me patiently, and his face grew serious while listening. It made me nervous because I had always witnessed him laughing and loving during these conversations. When I finished, he said, "it is alright that you are going through this, and it can be very natural to feel frustration and disappointment when you do not get answers to your questions."

"You are on the right track," he continued. Still, there is no need to chase the answers now but wait for them to come to you and soon, life will take you through those pathways and to people where you will find your answers. It will happen in an extraordinary way when life's secrets start opening to you. Still, everything will fit together in your life, and you will be surprised that it was so simple, and you took so much time to understand it, but there is no need to feel bad about it because it was not your time, and you were not ready for it."

He paused for a few moments (maybe, he was connecting with himself to find the correct phrases to guide me) and then smiled and continued, "you are still too young to understand this, and you have your whole life to enjoy. Right now, you are very young, and you should enjoy your childhood and student life. Once you grow up, many of these questions will guide you on where to go and what to do. Then you will get your answers slowly, so wait, be calm and patient, stop thinking about it for the time being, and enjoy what is in front of you."

"What do you think?" he asked.

I took a long deep breath and felt as though a ton of weight had lifted off my shoulders. I answered, "I agree, and I will follow what you have just advised."

Everything felt resolved, and after many years, I understood how he silently introduced the perception of time and space into my head. I understood him validating me, my anxiety, my curiosity and, at the same time, postponing it for the future so that I could enjoy the present moment.

Sometimes I wonder if my father was a magician or a natural hypnotist who understood so much about the mind, which he later explained through his years of meditation practice and working and understanding with the mind. So, here I am, like father, like son. The concept of being "now and here" refers to time and space because if I look back, I remember not worrying about tomorrow even though I had many challenging times while travelling to different countries. I was able to move away from those problems to be resolved in future when their time would come and separate myself from them and enjoy this very present moment.

I learnt that whenever possible, I needed to become aware that my life is of three seconds: the second which is left, the second which is this very moment, and the second which is coming. Further, I have no control over what has happened and equally no control over what will happen. The only reality is this very moment, and even previous and future seconds accompanying this very second cannot be that worthwhile. I can always, at this moment, select how I want to live it if I wish to be sad or happy. I can exert my right to live and enjoy this moment fully, or I can choose to be sad and cry. The freedom to choose and move between polarities (good or bad) and to have control over it can be one of the main tasks of living a life as a complete human being. Living in the present moment with the awareness of now and here without any distraction makes polarities secondary to you and your yearnings. There should be a direct connection and understanding partnership between you and your inner self.

It reminds me of an epic tale of Buddha, who shared this story with his disciples about living a life in that very second in between death. He narrated this story:

"Once upon a time, a man in a jungle was chased by a hungry lion. After running among the trees, he found a tree to climb on, and within a few moments, he climbed up to a safe height that the lion could not reach. He was so scared and tired of running for his life just to escape the hands of death.

After taking some deep breaths of relief and calming himself down, he felt less anxious and waited for the lion to go away so that he could get back home. The lion, however, continued to make unsuccessful attempts to climb the tree and at last sat down at the bottom of the tree, looked up at the man with frustration and made desperate roars.

Recovering his breath and senses, the man, with relief, started looking for alternatives to escape. While looking around, suddenly, he felt some movements on the upper part of the tree. When he looked up, he noticed a giant python was rapidly approaching him from the upper part of the tree.

He was caught between death and mixed feelings of panic, dread, and terror; his body trembled. Looking around desperately to find an escape, he anxiously caught sight of some fruit within his reach. He plucked the fruit and anxiously put it into his mouth, finding it to be surprisingly tasty.

He could not help but exclaim, "mmm, what delicious fruit!" and for that very second, he forgot his fear of death that was quickly advancing towards him. He completely surrendered himself to that very moment of delighting in the deliciousness of the fruit and forgot about the lion, python, and his dread.

Buddha explained, "for that very second, he forgot about death and lived a complete life in that very second."

After listening to the story, the disciples felt mesmerized by the enlightened intelligence of Buddha and wondered about the lessons hidden in the epic tale.

Wow, such a deep story and yet how simple it is! It beautifully narrates the importance of living a complete life in that very second and that very place. I found it so inspiring, touching and awakening. How has it helped you to understand yourself?

My father taught me how to meditate when I was four years old. It started with the mindfulness of breathing exercises and their use in various situations, followed by more profound visualization techniques. It helped me during some overwhelming situations, especially when I attracted bullies everywhere during my student life. Nevertheless, I was able to separate physical pain from mental pain.

Thus, I understood the power of the mind and its functions on a deeper level, and the seed to connecting with the source started growing enormously, which later came true when I had my whole life therapy process to get my license to work with Integrative Therapy of in-depth psychology from

Germany. I realized how I got my mother's anxiety when I was in the womb.

I felt what my father felt when I was in the womb. How are family traits and parents' desires transferred into a baby's womb, and how essential and indispensable is it to feel loved and accepted to live a healthy whole (complete) for the rest of my life? It helped me become one with myself, and I understood most of my life event's origin, whether it was suffering or happiness, was in me, and I started taking full responsibility for my life.

An ordinary person may suffer between good and evil, and maybe, his whole life is spent fighting between right and wrong or imagining situations that should, would or could have happened; consequently, his feelings alternate between guilt, regret, or shame, causing him to live less happily than he ought to. This is the leading cause of many unhealthy choices and decisions, forcing the unconscious psychic to take pathological conclusions about future mental or physical diseases.

Today, decades after following my father's advice, I realized that many of my questions have been answered, and my capacity to live in the present has grown enormously. I do not feel that anxious quest for answers; instead, I enjoy my life as much as possible. I suffer, I feel sad, I feel happy, and I enjoy life like every other human being. Still, my capacity to understand myself, my emotions, thoughts, and my subconscious responses to situations and experiences are far greater than before. I know that they will continue to grow with time as I journey through my life, just as everyone else.

My book "The need for disease" is the continuation of the pathway I chose with the support of my father, and whether you believe it or not, "Your disease or health is directly connected to your capacity of living Now and Here."

I am so grateful to all the people who have been a part of my journey, especially my parents, Raghu Nath Mehra and Darshi Mehra, and my friends and teachers, Dr. Jose Villalba and Dr. Werner J. Meinhold.

I am also eternally grateful to my wife Tatiana for her continuous unconditional support and love, and my biggest inspirations are my two daughters, Anisha Mehra, and Ambar Mehra.

*"Love brings me into existence,
and existence surrounds me with love."*

Atul Mehra

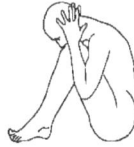

Chapter 1
The Origin of Human Consciousness

Pregnancy does not start from conception but rather when the mother imagines the first idea of having a baby and then sharing the idea with her husband/future father of the baby. Their conversations and decisions about having a baby start to influence the life of a forthcoming baby. The baby can also be influenced by the environment where Mom and Dad want the baby to take birth. Is it a stressful environment or a healthy environment? Would baby feel depressed, rejected, or sad because the relationship between parents is so stressful, riddled with arguments, creating sad, anxious, and depressing experiences? Would the baby feel happiness, joyness, acceptance and unconditional love because Mom and Dad love and support each other and hence create a peaceful environment?

Mother and baby relationship is one of the most important relationships in life. That is the part which welcomes us to join the human race on this planet. In fact, this is the base of all relationships in the future. Whatever the mother feels, does, hears, imagines, and thinks becomes the basis for the baby to interpret and bring to the rest of his life experiences. Mother and baby share the same body at first, as well as thoughts, emotions, sensations, and experiences. As mother is the one in the "driver's seat" throughout her pregnancy, it leaves the baby no choice but to feel what mother feels. The Mother's life is also directly influenced by her husband and her parents, as well as all others who occupy an important role in her or the baby's life. Any conditions imposed on the baby from his parents or from other influential people in the mother's life can also affect the future life of the baby. If people have expectations (conditions of acceptance) in the form of gender, colour of eyes, hair colour or skin tone, then they have the capacity to create trauma during pregnancy especially if the unborn does not meet those conditions as created by parents, especially by the mother.

Many scholars and researchers in birth psychology do not give any importance to the period lived by the baby before conception. In fact, there might be less than a handful of people talking about the period before conception because for most of us life starts when the baby takes birth, some of us now have started understanding the importance of intrauterine life from conception but my 21 years of research working with thousands of clients have taught me to understand the importance of the period lived by baby even before conception. The period before conception consists of three parts. First, the sperm carries the information of accepted or rejected child from father, second the ovum or information coming from the mother's side, and third at the time when the soul descends into the body. The conception is the completion of that triad, which is the information coming from the father, the mother and the purpose of the soul which inhabits the body. This is the greatest influence on the baby's life.

The simple feeling of acceptance or rejection can change the whole trajectory of baby's life and it can be the beginning of the rest of his life. Repetition of rejection or something similar can create malignant impregnation in baby's formation and become the cause of inviting a multitude of continuous unhealthy events in his life. A baby feels what mother feels. Mother's feelings for the baby are the first ever lived experiences of his life and they direct and guide the rest of his life. I would like to explain it with an example, let us say a mother wants to have a baby with blue eyes and blonde hair, and desires that he grows up to become a doctor. If the baby fulfills those conditions, then he is accepted by the mother and his life would be satisfactory and pleasant. On the other hand, if he does not fulfill these conditions, then he feels rejected by his mother, and now where there should be an unconditional love of mother, there is not. This means that if the baby does not feel loved unconditionally and accepted by the mother, then he will try to fill it with something else, maybe a pathology which can be any disorder or disease that prevents him from living his life as a "whole". He would live his life to fill that black hole, his true purpose of life is lost, and he would go around feeling unworthy, looking for validation and pleasing others. Do you think that you or someone you know has not lived a satisfied life, but has tried to fill the emptiness with things such as a successful profession, or another person, substance abuse, a hobby, or something else?

Let me clarify my point. This does not mean at all that all parents act this way intentionally or that they are responsible for their child's unhappiness and sadness. No, thinking or feeling that way is completely invalid and wrong. In fact, no one is to blame for this because first of all, they were not aware that this was happening and secondly, they also learnt it from their parents unconsciously when they did not have a rational mind. This is the same example as when a child learns his very first language in early age, he never thinks to challenge his parents about what they are teaching him or whether it is right or wrong; but as an adult, he can use his analytical mind to interpret a new language or reject learning it. If we must hold someone responsible for starting this whole phenomenon, then let us put the blame squarely on Adam and Eve from the Bible because as the story goes, they were the first man and woman who became parents.

Parents always love the best way they can because it is natural and they always do, or maybe they just could not love for whatever reason and rejected their child. Rejection can also be a way to connect with parents because underneath it, love is hidden. No matter what, either way you need to make peace with them in your heart otherwise it is always going to affect your life directly or indirectly. In order to accept yourself you need to accept your parents as they are, without wanting to change them.

The basis of our security and existence depends upon the love, acceptance and touch we feel in our intrauterine life. This further forms the foundation of our existence and of a balanced life. The physical and mental characteristics are transferred from parents to children in the form of biological and emotional information, including desires, inspiration, fears, happiness, frustration, expectations, etc. Nevertheless, there is no such thing as 100% acceptance, nor is there such a thing as 100% shortfall in a person's life. Hidden beneath that neurotic mask there is always an adequately healthy but unrecognized part of the self. The basis of our lifetime is created with the intrauterine processes lived by us during the gestational nine months. The development of our eighteen senses is just the beginning, and our experiences in our mother's womb are set to determine our future. All the information in every second is being recorded.

All experiences lived by the mother are lived by the baby also. Those experiences, irrespective of whether they are good or bad, are now a natural way of connecting with the mother. In his future life, the baby needs to either live or attract the same situations that he experienced during his intrauterine life because this is now his unconscious way of connecting with his mother.

If a baby does not develop the healthy contents of intrauterine life period such as unconditional love and acceptance, then he will try to seek them in subsequent or posterior periods but since he cannot find them there because other periods have their own healthy content then his life can be nothing but to fill the emptiness which he has to carry for rest of his life.

For example, If the mother does not think that the most important thing for her child in pregnancy is to give her love without any conditions (which is the corresponding and appropriate content) because the child feels what the mother feels. If the child does not receive this content or message, then he does not receive the imprint that he is accepted without condition. And the mother, of course, as she herself did not have/clearly live this feeling or experience of unconditional acceptance from her mother, transmits to the child her own life experience; but this is not an ill-intention on the part of the mother because she does not know that she is doing it. Then this child in his future life, just like his mother is going to try to fill the void she made. To fill the void that she also feels, the mother will try to feed the child very well.

This feeding transmits the message "I love you" to the child. In fact, this is not feeding and at the same time it does not fill the void of acceptance, thus the two phases are not filled. In a therapeutic process everything needs to be accepted and validated because there is no fake content. Behind the neurotic mask there is always the correct healthy content. There is no 100% deficit in a patient who has come to the consultation.

This is the subconscious mind which conveys the affection. So, when the mother in her own life story as a child learned that food created trust in her relationship with her mother, but love was untrustworthy because her mother might say "if you do this again, I won't love you", then love was not a reliable thing, but feeding was a reliable thing, then she takes the food to meet the demand for love and acceptance. The mother should have learned it in the same way. But we are not trying to look for who is responsible (as clarified before), but our idea is to reveal unconscious malignant patterns working underneath which take hold of our life by creating a pseudo security of being loved.

So, we have both phases without the healthy content or experience they should have, and we also have a food disorder. Later, this woman becomes an adult and develops problems, overeats because it is something reliable and provides her with security; but in reality, it is not a problem with food, but it was generated further back, in the search for unconditional love and acceptance.

The idea is neither not to eat at all, nor to create a fixation with food because every fixation is a disease. The main task here is that the person eats to nourish and for taste and this is a healthy response to food.

In order to understand this in a deeper way, I will use an example from the famous German poet, Goethe, who, in one of his poems, said, "if the first button of the shirt is placed into a wrong buttonhole, then all other buttons will be wrongly placed." The intrauterine life is the base of our life. It is the foundation of a house upon which the remainder of our life's building will be constructed. We need to know the symbolism so we can find in earlier stages earlier content. With this example of the buttons and the buttonholes, it is seen that this is very simply explained because we have a wrong button on each buttonhole, so no buttonhole is well buttoned.

During difficult times when both mother and baby feel the pain of rejection, guilt, or abandonment, mother can understand and rationalize these feelings and she has a capacity to separate herself from them; however, the baby cannot understand the nature of what he is experiencing. He does not yet have a rational brain to grasp the significance of his feelings. The child lives in a state of deep hypnosis for up to first three years of his life. The development of the analytical mind starts later than that. These painful intrauterine experiences may become transformed and expressed later as sentiments of worthlessness, guilt, seeking attention, pleasing others, or lacking self-love.

If a baby experiences continuous situation of conditional love, rejection, and life-threatening circumstances in his intrauterine life, then his life is more likely to suffer more opposition than those who have experienced more pleasant situations.

Everything we need, yearn for or desire is reduced to a connection of love. On the surface this sounds simplistic, but it is extraordinarily difficult because it is not just a want of love, but rather a continuous effort towards total and unconditional love that we seek from the moment we come into existence. Living a conditional intrauterine life means not being able to live and integrate healthy conditions of acceptance. Every life has a right to exist by the mere fact of being. Generally, we do not experience this well and therefore, we do not firmly establish security in life or a state of being that leads us to unconditional acceptance. The lack of acceptance, conscious or subconscious, creates deficiencies and anxieties that are then transmuted to future life conditions. A mother who transmits her anxiety onto the baby has learned this from her mother. In such conditions any sound therapy would neither generate guilt nor would it change the past conditions; instead, it would aim to lead the client towards acceptance with a holistic understanding.

The emotional stresses felt during this period generate a record of memorized reactions for rest of his life. As a developing human, he creates the neuronal-specific connections between the origins of his reactions and future events, which he will slowly but continually strengthen.

Investigation shows that depression and intrauterine fears create certain disturbances in the immune system, synapses, and the receptors of neurotransmitters, and in some cases within the brain structure. The cerebral cortex of the baby is thicker and is better equipped to learn quickly and has a highly developed intelligence, if his mother was privileged enough to live in a healthy environment where calmness, playing games, singing, and patting prevailed.

The experiences recorded during emotional traumas persist in an indelible way and may affect the cells and its functions. They remain hidden within the limbic system—the storehouse of our archaic emotional memory. This area is not naturally accessible to our developed consciousness. These stored impressions are responsible for multiple disturbances within our hormone and immune secretions. Stressful events stimulate these symbolic shortfalls, creating physical and mental discomfort, depression or even disease.

The basic anxieties borne out of rejection ensure that these rejected parts of the personality are routed and suppressed into the unconsciousness. Here they reside and become the roots of self-injurious and self-destructing psychosomatic disease. The "bad" or deficient parts of the personality can turn into malignant disease.

Disease is simultaneously an expression of trauma as well as of the security of existence (being) through which the person expresses himself. Insisting on removing these deficient parts of personality could cause malignancies through morbid metastasis. When the Intrauterine phase is disturbed, we cannot perceive life as an expression of the essence, and therefore, it exists with complete right and security by itself.

A great majority of diseases and disturbances that appear to be related to one or more of the early development periods have their origin (or the first buttonhole) in the Intrauterine phase. The phase where disturbance is generally found shows the intent to compensate the lack of basic existential security. If the baby did not feel the experience of initial acceptance, he will use the rest of his life to fill this lack, but as this is not the respective buttonhole to that button, he will never resolve the feeling of not having received it at its due time. For example, even though I can do everything, I am never satisfied.

If the moments of birth are problematic, then it means that already there were problems during pregnancy. If there is a premature delivery or if the baby does not want to take birth at this time, then there has to be a reason behind it.

There are other thirteen more important senses, besides the common five we have always known. For example, the sense of warmth which already exists and plays a significant role in the intrauterine phase, as the development of this sense gives the feeling of warmth, the symbol of love.

"The soul of disease is the same as the soul of health."

Atul Mehra

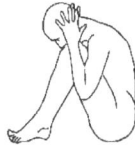

Chapter 2
Health and Disease

What is health? "Disease or No Disease," is that the question? Since the time we take birth to the moment when we die, we go in-between the states of wellbeing and sickness. We feel happy when we are healthy and feel sad when we are sick. Although these two uncomplicated words are unmistakable to understand, they simultaneously take on a different meaning when we try to understand them on an unconscious or deeper level. It becomes the base for realizing that everything is connected to the life we have been living.

Human beings are social by nature. Like most species on our planet, it is profitable to live in community and to follow its rules; but sometime those rules become so suffocating that they begin to influence our daily activities and lead to stress, sickness, physical, mental, or spiritual ailments. The society gives more importance to the "healthy ones" and looks at them from a different point of view than from the "sick ones." The society's needs and demands, diagnosis, treatment plans, how the family and oneself feel about being healthy or sick, all directly influence decisions related to health and disease. If we examine them carefully, we find that they are not very simple to understand.

Who is healthy? In fact, this is very difficult to understand because health is perceived as an absence of disease. Who has never been to a doctor or ever been carefully examined? Since the moment we are conceived to the moment we die, our body goes through millions of physical, mental, and spiritual processes which are critical for the development, adaptation, and survival of our human species.

In order to understand its deep interpretation of the states of health and disease, Dr. Werner Meinhold invites us to examine a case of a 42-year-old man who always felt very well and has been very efficient in his work. While he was working one day at his office, he unexpectedly experiences a strong pain in his chest and breaks out into a cold sweat. He is taken into the emergency where the tests revealed that he suffered a myocardial infarction (heart attack). In this case there is no doubt that he had always been healthy but now he is sick.

Do numerous questions arise about his health in your mind? Would he survive the heart attack? If yes, then did he recover and return to his work and previous productivity? Would he, his family or his coworkers have the confidence that he has recovered completely? Now the question remains, "is he really healthy?"

The modern diagnosis of a heart attack generally emphasizes a resolution of the physical symptoms, but it does not include recovery at the mental and spiritual levels. The true meaning of health or disease becomes complex when we take into consideration the psychic and spiritual level of the patient.

Many of us know that heart attacks are linked to smoking, being overweight, nutritional deficiencies, lack of exercises and chronic stress, among other contributing factors. Living with one or more of these factors increases the risk of a heart attack.

The most surprising fact is that he reacted the same way as do a vast majority of heart attack patients and that is as if his life was not at all important or as if he did not know anything about it. His risk factors intertwined: he had chronic stress and his smoking habit served as a tranquilizer (symbolically mother breast feeding), as well as uncontrolled eating led to being overweight which was exacerbated by a lack of exercise, relaxation, or recreational activities.

What were the causes beneath all of this? What led him to this? We need to take into consideration his external causes such as professional obligations, social status, standard of living and all insubstantial values that are not the essential nature of a human being.

Without doubt life is the only base of our existence and rest everything else depends upon it. We need to know the deeper meaning of life and how life should be lived "correctly?" We can discuss that or maybe we can give recommendations to others based on those criteria.

The most common philosophy of life claims that fundamentally every life is worth living without any special conditions. To be able to live true to this statement we need to respect life and live with a loving attitude towards ourselves, releasing the possibilities of self-harming and self-destructive behaviour.

Now this brings us to the question, "When did this disease begin in this patient?" "Did the self-harm begin even as he felt healthy and productive, or did it begin only when he suffered a heart attack?"

If we look at this case from this point of view, then his disease would be a call to attention to stop his self-destructive, pathological behaviour. During his stay in intensive care in hospital, he was forced to suspend his self-aggressive activities and thus became healthier than before. However, after his discharge from the hospital once being pronounced as "healthy", he would fall back into his habitual self-harming behaviour, which would lead to him becoming sick again.

Modern medicine only provides treatments that remove the symptoms of disease, but do not address the deeper problems that are rooted at the unconscious level. Let us imagine a treatment which makes unconscious conscious as Jung said and he discovers the unconscious motives which led him to create a heart attack. He discovers that he has forced himself to achieve maximum productivity due to his unconscious fear of not being accepted. Thus, while this patient appeared to be externally healthy, he was, in fact, the exact opposite internally due to his pathological behaviour that do not respect the essential and fundamental foundations of life.

This further leads to the consequence that this patient cannot live a satisfactory life, nor can he overcome his unconscious doubts about being accepted in his own right. Due to this he adds an unconscious tendency to punish himself which he expresses through self-destructive behaviour before and after having a heart attack.

This type of connection, along with life circumstances and the psychological and spiritual influences of life, such as the ones we discussed in the example of the heart patient, can be discovered working with the unconscious mind in most of the cases. This also applies to those diseases that are caused by bacteria and virus etc.

Our immune system is connected to our unconscious psyche which decides whether a contagious disease should appear or not.

Other forms of sicknesses go through our limbic system within our brain which transforms the psychic impulses directly in vegetative regulation and in the endocrine glands, further creating 'psychosomatic diseases."

The common criteria are that the disease should disappear as soon as possible, so that everything can go back as it was before. This is wrong. Humans are not biological machines who are affected by an alteration of the bio-mechanical function; we need to gain a deeper sense of understanding and its origin.

That is why a medication or treatment which takes care of a human being at all levels (i.e., physical, emotional, and spiritual) should not be affected by the same symptoms of the patient who tries to cure them and only settles the obvious damages like we have seen in the previous example of the heart patient. It is not enough to have success in restoring the physical and intellectual functions in a human; we also need to be aware of the hidden connections that exist within the emotional and spiritual levels, and emphasize a total, holistic diagnosis followed by integral therapy. Then the disease is accepted and recognized as part of one's life history that contains a valid and worthwhile meaning.

Therefore, being sick in our example meant a pathway to heart attack, but now we can bring greater, more complete well-being, which is discovered by the patient himself, leading one to being more kind to himself and to the loved ones around him.

Health and disease from this holistic point of view are abstract concepts that only become clear when they become the subjective experience of each individual carrying its own significance. It is obvious that a simple physical diagnosis, a corresponding label, and the treatment of a disease can only point to a fraction of the individual's subjectivity.

It is important to highlight that a common physical exam can be combined with an inventory of the psyche and the influences of environment (bio-psychosocial anamnesis) to form basis for holistic therapy; but it is not sufficient because within the phases of one's history of life many offensive conditions are repressed within the unconscious and cannot be discovered with anamnesis without conscious hypnosis.

The unconsciousness is this additional level which is most important for understanding the sick person and it can only be made conscious through depth psychology with conscious hypnosis because it can travel into deeper levels than typical psychoanalysis does.

Finally, I would like to mention the other aspect of the question about health and disease which is particularly important for the mentally ill people, and their family and friends.

"How does the mentally ill person react and how does his environment react when he is ill?"

The person who is sick can experience many emotions: pity, reproach, scorn, defensive attitude, fear, disgust, isolation etc. These can originate from outside or from within. It is relatively easy to observe that those with a mental illness are met with a lack of understanding and with scorn (sometimes they utter these themselves). It is widely known that will-power does not get rid of the symptoms such as fear, obsession, or depression. We cannot possibly eliminate gallstones with will-power, but in this case, one would not think to counsel the patient to expel it.

It is still more difficult to explain the fact that many times we fear those who are mentally ill, and due to this they lose friendships. As if their illness is an infectious and dangerous process! We know that those with a mental illness are prone to less violent acts and there is no possibility to get infected in comparison to the "healthy ones." Thus, there is no reason to walk away from these illnesses in comparison to the diseases that present themselves at the physical level.

The psychoanalytical research on this phenomenon deserves an explanation. The fear of becoming infected has an unconscious basis. The mentally ill person symbolically expresses his conflicts through his symptoms. The recognition of these symbols by him acting as an observer for himself can awaken in him the unconscious fear that similar conflicts can be triggered.

This forces the persons near him to react by protecting himself in the form of fear, which in fact is the protection in front of himself (it means his unconscious transference to the person diagnosed as sick). As a second step, he also physically separates like a symbolic form of moving away from his own fears.

Something similar happens with the social and political deficit of acceptance towards the mentally ill and also for psychotherapy. It is completely opposite to the acceptance extended to the physically ill, as well as to the methods used for treatment such as medication and surgery, etc. A good example of this is the fact that higher costs for physical treatments are covered by medical insurance providers in comparison to the lower cost coverage provided for psychotherapy treatments (In Canada this means that 95% of therapies are done by medication, medical devices, and surgery in comparison to 5% for physiotherapy or psychotherapy).

Therapies based on depth psychology -- which in the long run are more successful and economical than long repetitive medical treatments -- do not have any collateral damaging effects. Other favourable argument is that when there are unknown mental or spiritual disorders, medical treatments cannot deal with them, but psychotherapy can treat and heal all ailments that are physical, mental, and spiritual.

The reason why fears and prejudices in bodily diseases appear weaker is because the unconscious causes of physical diseases are more difficult to decipher than the psychic level and therefore are less frightening. The translation of the psychic to the physical level has been written, so to speak, as a code that cannot be easily understood. I can hardly recognize the repressed psychic components.

The physical illness appears as something strange, as a thing that has occurred without any contribution of its own and something that must be eliminated. Physical illnesses are an exception in which there are fears of their own, conscious, or unconscious, for example AIDS (sexual and mortal fears) or cancer (fear of "bad" and death). In this case the corresponding unconscious projection or identification also leads to withdrawal, which is explained by a fear of infection.

A more extensive understanding of health and illness is probably one of the most important steps in the way to be kinder to oneself and for the recovery of health. Another important step would be to have a more open concept in the current system of health, which is in a system of "disease management" and introduce a more holistic system which honors and validates the complex reality of the human being.

"It's no measure of health to be well adjusted to a profoundly sick society."

Jiddu Krishnamurti

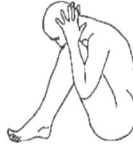

Chapter 3
Do We Live in a Sick Society?

We live in a world where success is an essential part of our life. People do not see us as who we are but how successful we have been in our life. Do you have a big house, a profession of the year or killer good looks? The simple fact of the matter is what matters most is" what is your worth?"

Society demands that we follow social rules and obligations, which is appropriate but only to the point that they should not dominate our lives. However, when these rules and obligations go out of control then some things in our life begin to change. Let us examine what is implied in this sentence:" If you are not efficient then you are worth nothing". Although this statement is not commonly heard in everyday life, its subtle message affects every area of our life. Do you fear that if you do not perform optimally in your job then you may be fired someday soon?

Mesmer believed that we live in a sick society. Efficiency has come to play an important role in our society because it leads to rewards and recognition. To be recognized or accepted is a basic human desire and leads to happiness. Unfortunately, this same strong desire to be recognized can lead us to create serious diseases such as cancer. The brain's emotive powers can trigger a disease as dangerous and life-threatening as cancer if this essential need to be recognized or accepted remains unmet during one's life.

Let me illustrate this postulation with an example. Let us suppose that the hidden message to be accepted has three conditions attached — I know that it sounds ridiculous to suggest this but for an individual who leads with his/her emotional brain, this can become a deeply impactful reality. A woman who has an enviable profession, a figure like a model, or be a natural blue-eyed blond has just completed the three neurotic conditions that she feels will gain acceptance from society, and then everything will line up perfectly in her life. However, if she does not fulfill these three conditions and fails to get that recognition, she will bear an additional pressure of having failed that will disturb her in everyday life. As a woman with a high sense of self-worth and self-acceptance, she knows and believes that it makes no iota of a difference whether she is blue-eyed or not and does not have an enviable job. She is secure in knowing that she has other finer qualities. Not every woman responds in the same way to this inner conflict. Some accept it, somewhat defeated, and will go through life feeling emptiness, but some others find ways to express it through a disease. Still others may live the rest of the life deciphering subconsciously how they should live, dyeing their hair various shades, go through costly procedures like liposuction to reduce extra weight or liposuction, or even hiring a coach or following a Guru to fill the emptiness of having a less than perfect life.

The need for acceptance is so deeply embedded into our subconscious mind since early childhood that it is certain that almost every one of us has experienced it. For example, when a child is behaving inappropriately and the mother disapproves, she might say "don't do it or.... else." She sends an indirect hidden message to the child that her love and acceptance of the child is bound with conditions. If you do this, then I will not love you or I will only love you if you are a humble and compliant son. She, in fact, sends a message that she will completely reject the child under certain conditions but ignore the part that is "doing". She completely ignores his other positive traits and qualities and rejects him/her as a whole. May perhaps she has learnt it from her parents or she in unaware of what message she is imparting; nevertheless, it happens more often than not. Although she has an abundance of love for her son or daughter, she bends to conform to social rules because it is very difficult to go against the herd. But what about the child in this example? He/she has two options: obey the mother or rebel. In order to comply, he has to stop the behaviour which is disliked by the mother. So, his unconscious mind divides the behaviour into small parts with the disliked part staying hidden perhaps for the rest of his/her life. This part remains hidden from the mother and the later substitutes of mother (such as relatives, friends, wife or husband, children or other significant adults), but eventually this part does not remain hidden and starts showing up in the form of anxiety, depression, or other mental disorder.

The second option of rebelling against the mother's wishes and continuing the misbehavior implies that he does not care for the mother's acceptance and love. However, the child continues that behaviour at the expense of sacrificing the mother's love and consequently feels an inner emptiness. Then, he looks for a substitute to fill this gaping void. As a literal example, let's say that the child goes to the kitchen, makes a sandwich, and eats it to fill the emptiness and feel some kind of relief. Mother's love is an abstract idea in contrast with the solid experience of eating a sandwich. Mother's love has been replaced by the sandwich, so every time he feels this emptiness, he will fill it with a sandwich (or other food). Sadly, this emptiness is a black hole, and the sandwich is simply a temporary solution. The more you eat, the less it satisfies. What kind of chaos will it take in his life to fill that black hole? This is not the end of it because his way of expressing his love towards his own children is by giving them food or sandwiches. In fact, we live in an oral society where it is commonplace to think and ask, "don't you love your kids, see how skinny they are, don't you feed them?" What does love has to do with food?

I was recently reading some shocking news where the headline screamed "Meghan's father accuses daughter of cheapening UK" s royal family." His father said in an interview that he believed Meghan was tossing away "every girl's dream." It's disappointing because she actually got every girl's dream. Every young girl wants to become princess and she achieved that and now she's tossing that away, for, it looks like she's tossing that away for money," he said. "They are destroying it, they are cheapening it, they're making it shabby ... They are turning it into a Walmart with a crown of it now. It is something that is ridiculous, they shouldn't be doing this." Thomas Markle said he did not expect Meghan to get in contact. "I can't see her reaching out to me, especially now ... or Harry for that matter, but I think both of them are turning into lost souls at this point," he said. (Published on Jan. 19, 2020, by Reuters Staff, reporting by Elizabeth Piper, Editing by Frances Kerry)

What do you think of this? I am sure it will help you to understand how deeply rooted we are in in social norms and conditions. What are your dreams and frustrations?

Now you can see how these hidden messages impact our lives. Many similar things happen not only for women but also for men, children, senior citizens, and even newborn babies or babies in utero. Everyone participates in this stressful race that has no end. The wildly popular Marilyn Monroe suffered this pain her entire life and the martial arts champion-actor Bruce Lee died at a young age from a mysterious affliction, perhaps borne in the unconscious mind. Today's stressful, demanding lifestyle pressures us into pleasing others to be recognized but sadly contributes to too many mental and physical disorders.

The question that arises is this: how do we exit this race of always striving, pleasing others and transcend our desires to live a better life? Now that this has been brought into your awareness, I hope that the next few chapters will help you to understand this on a much deeper level.

*"Normal norms create neurosis that is
why we live in Normosis."*

Atul Mehra

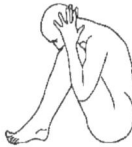

Chapter 4
The Normosis

I wish to make a special mention of the word taught to me by my friend and teacher Dr. Werner Meinhold because it made complete sense to understand the hidden conditions that lead to anxiety, depression, and other disorders. He used the word **Normosis** to explain the distorted Intrauterine content that results from a search for basic Intrauterine content in subsequent phases in the midst of an environment that is impregnated with the same distortion.

For example, when the baby could not live within a heathy context of unconditional love and acceptance in his mother's womb then he attempts to seek them in other phases of life which are already acculturated with same shortfalls. The individual unconscious need for this search and the conditions of acceptance imposed by the family and society, then are impregnated through the family environment, the parents and the mother into the baby that is being developed in womb. These are the neurotic conditions of acceptance that, due to their generalization, seem "normal." it means that those conditions look normal but in fact they are pathologies. For example, A neurotic statement would be *if you are inefficient, then you are worth nothing.* Although nobody says it out loud, we feel it instinctively and fear it every day in our lives, whether consciously or unconsciously. It is normal and it is an abstract norm. It forms the word Normosis, which combines the words *Norms* and *Neurosis.* It refers to anything that looks normal but is in fact a disease laden with hidden meanings. We live in normotic conditions with normotic symptoms. This model also helps us to bring into awareness our cultural pathologies. These pathologies are more serious because they are not recognized, it is normal to have them because they seem healthy.

It means that the patient and therapist are a part of same pathology, and the only healthy thing is to be a symptom of the disease. The patient creates symptoms which do not agree with Normosis, then, as both therapist and patient, being in the same neurotic condition, try to make that disagreed symptom disappear, the disease looks for another pathway to show up.

In the analytical phase of development, the Normotic symptom is that life is worth living only if you are efficient and producing results. Generally, tradition health systems in countries treat patients through therapies enough to make the person functional but does not proceed to do therapeutic work to find deeper issues that are working beneath to cause illnesses.

The word Normotic implies that it is psychotic, but it is accepted as the norm and thus everyone follows it. In other words, it is like psychosis, which is a serious illness, but the whole population has it, so it is widely accepted and becomes routine as opposed to being considered pathological in nature. For example, in India giving a birth to a boy is considered to be a blessing and giving birth to a girl is scorned and perceived as a curse; this leads parents to use ultrasounds and other modern methods to find out the gender of their baby before birth so that they could decide whether to keep the boy if it is a boy, or to terminate the pregnancy if it is a girl. How pathetic!

A boy is widely viewed as an asset, a future breadwinner and caregiver who will look after his parents when they become old. A girl, on the other hand, is seen as a liability, as parents are often pressured to pay dowries when their daughters marry.

Also, in India, it is considered son's pious obligation to take care of his parents, but no such expectation is placed upon daughters. After marriage, a daughter is usually regarded as a member of her husband's household and is generally expected to take care of her in-laws, but not her parents. A son is also the one who will carry the family name for progeny. I have resolved many cases where my female clients felt worthless because they did not give birth to a boy. In other cases, the boys were given more preference and freedom than girls which resulted in different mental and physical disorders.

After having a closer look at this social norm, the economics here is pretty straightforward. It's the culture that's to be blamed. The system as it stands today rewards the birth of a son, while penalizing the birth of a daughter. This is what I call the Normotic Effect.

This example has two main characteristics, first, a majority agrees with the idea that having a boy is fortunate because he will take care of the parents; secondly, since it is a strong social, they have to follow it otherwise they might be ostracized or looked down upon. This gives a rise to inner conflict that says what should we do versus what others want us to do.

It is also important to observe how regional languages describe much of the symbolism of that culture and its normotic diseases, their existence over all centuries, always normotic disease, true mental epidemics. For example, Emperor Charlemagne Saxony instituted the death penalty against burning alleged witches, but later witches were being burned at the stake. In this example, we do not see an adequate development of mind, in fact, in previous centuries they were much sicker in their mind.

Today, we are in our own normosis with our normotic symptoms and diseases. To look for these diseases we need to exit our cultural group because within these norms seem normal within the group.

For example, cellular phones are a current and contemporary normosis because through them we connect and communicate with each other. However, for deeper communication we need to meet face-to-face and connect with each other. The paradox of "the cellular is the technical communication that excludes": it brings distant people closer but excludes us from communicating with the one who is sitting beside us. It actually removes the need for contact.

Thus, the technical communication is in analytical phase here because of its symbolism and with the danger that all communication goes through computers. For example, people who can do their work on computers at their home office instead of going to their workplace office. They have no connection with others and become more disconnected and lonelier.

In the cultural phase where we are presently, we apply the technical approach to fulfill and correct the intrauterine need for contact. We try to correct the deficits of the intrauterine phase through analytical means but that requires us to be perfect and to create perfection (Analytical phase symbolism) in order to gain acceptance and unconditional love (Intrauterine Phase) from those who act as a substitute-mother.

Everything alive is like a wave, but this is a wave of Probability, it is not fixed otherwise it would not be life. We do not know about the wave while we are on the wave, we only know it by observing it, but this is also difficult because being on the wave means that we can only be at one point in it.

The present day normosis is suffocating our lives. Instead of breaking free from it, we are becoming a part of it and that leads us to creating anxiety, ADHD, depression, mood disorders, psychosis, and other mental illnesses. Many of us do not know about it and those who know just ignore it because most of the time is spent in making a living, paying taxes and other expenses, and generally busy living a life. Every day we have less and less time for ourselves and more time to fulfill the Normotic demands. Even young children are being introduced to Normosis and are socialized to accept it.

We lead normotic lives and yet we all know deep down inside our hearts that the future of humanity is in grave danger because of it. Can covid-19 be a way to show us that we are living a normotic life?

"The unconscious mind of a man sees correctly even when conscious reason is blind and impotent."

Carl Jung

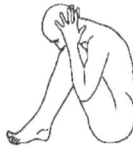

Chapter 5
The Unconscious Resistance

Are you unconsciously resistant to give up your disease?

This question seems very odd to us because it creates a question in our minds that why someone would not like to give up his disease. It creates some confusion, fear, and disturbance within our rational faculty, causing us to want to discard it by thinking that it is some kind of a joke or a strange question to ask.

The battle between health and disease is essentially a lifelong quest.

Unconscious resistance refers to a psychological pattern of creating situations that prevents a person from becoming completely healthy, instead he creates obstacles to health because his disease somehow serves as a pseudo security blanket for him at an unconscious level. The root of any disease is deeply anchored within the patient himself. In other words, every disease is created by the person himself and since no disease is created consciously, it means that all diseases are unconscious and so are the obstacles created by the patient. The origin of disease come from within deepest psychological layers for which our logical and analytical mind seeks to find explanations. Let us say a general anxiety may be created by the person himself when he was around 2 or 3 years old, and it has served as a form of protection from the outside world. The analytical mind rationalizes it by analyzing the situations of recent events created anxiety where he had a heated argument with his spouse and interpret that as its origin.

Would it appear illogical to say that someone would not like to become healthy, especially if they are suffering tremendously as a result of having depression? Then why would he want to create obstacles to oppose the therapeutic process of healing? Who would not like to live a healthy life?

It is difficult to answer all these questions because we need to explore, understand, and process the malignant patterns hidden beneath the surface, causing uncomfortable situations in a person's life. One would unconsciously want to preserve his illness and create obstacles in the therapeutic process because his disease is a mask through which he is expressing his hidden conflicts, while at the same
time it serves as a protection against discovering and processing those psychic wounds and fears repressed in the unconscious basement.

Research shows that it is easier for a person to create cancer than confront his basic fears connected with his essence of being a human. It means the experiences lived in the mother's womb or in early childhood are connected with deep fears, but they are locked up in the unconscious basement. Confronting these repressed fears, opening those shut-off memories abruptly or accessing them too rapidly can create psychosis, depression, suicide ideation or cause the patient to discontinue the therapeutic process.

According to Meinhold, these resistances are expressed as "masked." In the critical periods of therapy, they can appear as, for example, unpleasant feelings against the therapy or the therapist, or doubt against his efficiency, a desire to interrupt or discontinue the therapy, delay and forgetting the session, etc. Also, falling in love with the therapist has many times an unconscious function of blocking the therapy.

Another frequent resistance is expressed through patient's tendency to read psychology books while continuing therapy or simultaneously consulting other analytic therapies or other therapists. This leads to the alleged ability to judge the therapist, but in reality, it is a stimulation of the resistance with the possibility of "not accepting" the unpleasant interpretations.

That is why many patients leave the therapeutic process when they feel pain or they do not want to access the memories which cause pain, choosing instead to simply move on without processing and integrating them. They look out for information on the internet or seek other therapeutic methods because they would rather remain in their comfort zone than work at processing their pain unconsciously.

In addition, unconscious resistance is also the reason for many people to reject the analytic therapy methods and seek other types of treatments where they can leave everything as it was before (and how they had first created the disease), because they only want to lose their symptoms quickly. This is one of the main reasons why we look for quick solutions. We opt for therapies which can give us fast relief and put us back to work as soon as possible. In fact, this results in a symptom shift which has been explained in detail in the chapter *What is symptom?*

Majority of the therapeutic process do not know the importance of unconscious resistance and use analytical methods to surpass the original content for which the disease or disorder was created. Many therapists are not even aware of unconscious resistance and unconsciously try to please their clients by creating conditions where patients experience temporary symptom relief and call it healing.

The appropriate therapeutic management of resistances is one of the most important tasks on the path to health. In every therapy arrangement (the agreement between patient and therapist on the modalities of therapy) the possibility of the appearance of resistances should be explained clearly and all patients should make a contract with themselves not to surrender when resistances are presented.

It is very important that more research be conducted, and information made available to the therapists and the clients to help them understand unconscious resistance because every therapeutic process aims to heal but it also simultaneously fires up one's unconscious resistance to heal.

"Integrate love as consciousness and not as an emotion."
"Love me or hate me either way, you are with me."
"Love as an emotion finds its balance in hate, separation, pain, or fear."

Atul Mehra

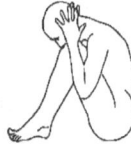

Chapter 6
Transference- The Unconscious Hook

I always held an idea with certainty that Transference and Counter-transference can be perceived as little more than a therapeutic process, but I was in for a huge surprise and when I learnt that most of our life is surrounded by transference and counter-transference. It helped make sense of many things in life and many of my own daily behaviours and questions began to receive their answers. I decided to add some great examples of transference and countertransference based on the research of my friend and teacher Dr. Werner Meinhold.

I am sure that it will arouse a curiosity about relationships around you, and maybe you will be able to resolve some eternal puzzles in your life and generate more understanding and peace with yourself.

The processes of transference exist in all intense relationships in everyday life and every therapeutic relationship as well. It makes us live situations where a person transfers or directs the sentiments or actions which stem from the past, it means, from the deficit childhood or in-womb experiences, onto a person or a situation of a present life with whom he has an emotional bond. It stands for the redirection of sentiments to a substitute. In this kind of communication, the ones involved are similar to the theatre actors who play specific roles learnt from their childhood. Nevertheless, they are under the illusion that what they feel and express belongs to their present reality. The opposite person frequently responds with his own role of transference (which comes from his own childhood deficit) which generally fits in our correspondence with the role of the other one. This process is known as Countertransference. In our culture there are many common deficit impregnations.

The Transference and Countertransference, or as I also call them "The Unconscious Hooks", do not happen at the conscious level. They are generally invisible because they take place at an unconscious level. This type of communication develops in a direct way, which means that in this system we cannot differentiate between who is an initiator or who is a receiver of the message as it happens simultaneously. From here, the singularity derives from the fact that in this system, there is no one to blame, since it is a direct exchange system where you cannot know who has started and who has answered. In every person we can normally find different type of strong mixed sentiments of transference, so it is not very easy to recognize them.

For example, the intense desire to be with the partner or the other one can be so intense, that every absence or unavailability can be perceived as an insult, offend, or wound. In this case this addresses to a transference of Intrauterine wish and sentiment, which come from the earliest infancy or before, when mother was absent or not sufficiently available. This deficit gets engraved on the subconscious mind of an adult, that is why, he unconsciously attempts to transfer the role of the mother to his/her partner. Entirely the same, this necessity of recovering the mother can never be satisfied with this method because the window of corresponding growth is closed, and he needs a very specialized therapeutic method to open it. I have resolved many similar situations with different clients simply explaining the process of transference and counter- transference. Many of them showed their remorse and wasting time, money and efforts finding solutions elsewhere, but at the same time they were amazed by how simple it was to blame his/her partner and once they realized the hidden patterns, their lives were changed for good.

How should a person live his life with his partner? Should he live with anxiety, belligerence, guilt, and domination? Of course, everybody knows the right answer, but we occasionally live out these undesirable situations.

A healthy relationship between two healthy adults should be lived without any feeling of transference as much as possible and that can only come if they are ready to understand that if you point someone with one finger there and three that are pointing at you. They have to be open, honest, understanding, and willing to accept and process the dark connections working underneath. The healthy relationship is also determined by their present internal and external situations.

Can you imagine a life of a person who does not have any neurotic impregnation? How would he react in case he gets any transference feelings from his spouse? Although, it is very uncommon to find a person who is living his life without any neurotic impregnation, but we can imagine that he would not get affected by the reaction of his own feeling and would consider them inadequate when he receives the feelings and reactions of transference from someone else.

Have you ever heard saying to someone "don't take it to your heart?" This sentence is a very good example of neurotic impregnation and at the same time it is trying to address the issue of the situation of the person that he may be going through some internal unconscious reaction or transference.

The other example of transference and countertransference can be seen in acrimonious relationships. The fights, heated arguments or caustic words occur frequently in these types of relationships often due to trivial matters. Here the transference has to be connected with analytical phase (development of reasoning or logical, analytical mind which is about 3-4 years old child brain). The adult in transference wants to sweep over his childhood situation where his efforts to impose were truncated, but this childhood void cannot be filled either because the fights between them repeat themselves over and over again. The aggressive behaviour is a conditional reflection.

The other objective of these aggressions can be that the contestant has learnt from his childhood that a bitter relationship is more important than a loving one because it was deficient in childhood. A popular joke states that a woman went to a priest to complain that her husband no longer loves her. When the priest asks her "how do you know?", she answers "because he does not hit me anymore."

I have experienced hundreds of sessions of couple therapy where the main issue has dealt with this type of acrimony or aggression. During regular counselling sessions when they argued it was nothing but a race to the present and an attempt to dominate the argument, to assert their own point of view and not let the other person speak. At times I allowed them to express their bitterness, during other times when it became too loud and resorted to name-calling, I had to intervene by standing in between them to stop them. I remember congratulating them for expressing themselves openly and bringing into awareness of how they connect with each other through rejection, arguments, and a lack of love. With experience, my way of explaining this and working to treat couples changed. I explained about transference and countertransference to them first, and then invited them to have individual sessions with me. I wanted them to understand the origins of their repetitive hidden patterns and malignant connections defining their relationships with their partner and thus understanding themselves better. Subsequently, it opened up the possibilities of understanding their partner better and on a much deeper level to enjoy the privileges offered by the unconditional love and live a more satisfying life than before.

Allow me to explain it with an example, when in a fighting relationship the patient no longer engages in previous aggressive behaviour from and wants to seek a peaceful solution. His partner may feel less received or welcomed than before because he does not want to argue anymore. As it has been already mentioned, transference feelings and behaviours are substitutes for basic needs, such as feeling of touch (better to receive blows than no contact). If the partner is sufficiently open and understanding, then he would not hesitate to ask for therapeutic help too.

The other types of transference are known as the complementary transferences. They represent the necessity of mutual transference and countertransference. Unfortunately, they can last for the whole life and the participants are not at all aware about the situations they are living, and it can happen between 2 or more people of a family or a group and so on. In fact, due to unfavourable circumstances, such as the loss of a partner (which can even be a dog) or of the couple, such system can be developed. If a substitute is not found, then, it can happen as a consequence that other person dies, for example of cancer.

When the partners of transference are separated, the former partners feel pain and generally reject each other. Even so, after the split they search again for a partner with similar characteristics (transferences). If that fails, a very serious mental or physical illnesses can appear. In this case the disease replaces the transferential partner.

Lamentably, in the event of the death of a transferential partner, the other can transfer this role to the dead person's memory. Now the transfer works even better since it is not in conflict with reality (sanctification of the dead). This effect is also known as the sanctification of historical characters.

As cited above, transference feelings are perceived as real, contemporary, and authentic, but their true origin remains unconscious. The transferences expressed physically are even more difficult to recognize because with this expression their psychic causes are even more hidden. In the example above, this could mean that the partner's desire for permanent presence is indirectly expressed through a bodily illness, which suggests the availability of the other (for example, taking care of the person). Here the caring partner often has a complementary transference attitude, for example, the so-called 'helper syndrome' (unhealthy desire to provide help to others, generally neglecting his own interests). On the contrary, the helper syndrome can also create in the other person the subconscious desire to get sick.

In addition to the common feelings of transference, there are also polarized transferences, in these cases he "idealizes" or "demons" to his partner with this transference, projecting his inner suppressed "ideals or evils."

When the person of transference is getting acquainted more closely, then the reality modifies its idealization and abandons the Prince Charming idea, observing him more closely, he stops becoming a prince and loses his charm. Materializing the relationship with the previously idealized person, a symbiotic union occurs. This has, therefore, the self-esteem deficit which had been trying to, fill, in the union with the prince, is proved as a deep bottomless pit which cannot be filled with anyone and with anything. Consequently, the union with the idealized partner cannot raise the person to the prince's level, but degrades him, lowering him to his own level. This is, by the way, the reason why stories and movies that tell idealized relationships end with the death of one or both participants (for example, Romeo and Juliet), or end the story with the well-known "happy ending" "which would be the beginning of the concrete couple relationship.

The transferential love relationships can be more lasting and "safer" when they have little probability to the real answers because their objects remain distant, such as movie or sports idols etc.

Surprisingly, instead of the transference of love, there can be a transference of identification, which is more or less conscious, generally with a person of the same sex. This can lead to paradoxical situations, in which, for example a soccer fan, who has nothing to do with sports, drinks beer sitting in front of a television, identifies himself with a high-class athlete, and worries about his victory. If his idol of transference loses the game, it can happen that he expresses his disappointment against the television and throws it out of the window. Such a transference to an idol clearly demonstrates him being out of reality in the transference situation.

It is equally absurd when a pensioner with rigid moral principles, living on a minimal monthly payment, buys magazines to find out the news of his rich and famous idols who live luxuriously and wildly on the money of the millions of poor people who admire them.

Thus, many industries profit with the romantic television soap operas and with the production of series of films with the themes of identification. Using the transference of identification fosters the illusion of a fantasy and "free" life, although, this freedom only consists in the selection of the program, film or TV series and nothing else.

Only this transference mechanism allows explanations for the surprising phenomenon that in some political systems a small minority of magnates are blatantly supported by the masses of whom they take advantage of.

Fortunately, transference also opens up exceptional possibilities for therapy. Transference is a ubiquitous condition in any therapeutic situation. As already brought up, each transference process includes a partial regression to childhood and with it a revival of the corresponding hypnotic states of this age.

In mild diseases, an "ideal" transference may be sufficient to promote self-healing processes. In serious diseases, a favourable transference situation is a good precondition for the acceptance of treatment measures and decisive for their success.

In the treatment based on in-depth psychology with conscious hypnosis by Dr Werner Meinhold, transference phenomena have an even more significant role. This is because the transference is already included through the hypnotic state of consciousness and thus connects with the pre-verbal phases of childhood and the extensive transference feelings pertaining to them.

In concert with the stimuli that trigger the transference processes at this basic level of hypnotic communication, there exists a form of telepathic connection between the patient and the therapist, corresponding to the original connection between mother and child (named as "archaic involvement"). This determines that this connection is facilitated not only by the spoken word or by body language, but also by the psychic processes carrying the transference. Therefore it is particularly important, in therapy, for the deep tuning of the therapist with himself and his therapeutic actions. Likewise, the basic necessity of having the broadest possible attitude of acceptance towards the patient cannot be met if he responds only with a technical knowledge towards this special and intimate level of therapy.

While working with in-depth psychology hypnotherapy, everything has to be carried out correctly, both externally and internally to promote the corresponding development.

The feelings that the therapist projects to the patient, in response to the patient's transfer to the therapist, are known as "countertransference." To prevent the therapist from unconsciously answering the patient's transferences with his own neurotic reactions, the school of in-depth psychology requires as an essential element of training where each therapist walk the path of whole life therapy process where he deeply works on himself to resolve his whole life issues starting from his present age and going backwards until conception.

"You just can't close the closet of the past."

Atul Mehra

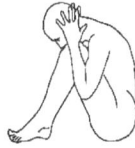

Chapter 7
Isn't it Better to Leave your Past in Peace?

Every day, one way or the other, I have witnessed people saying or suggesting to others, "just move on or "forget it, it is the part of the past."

It also surprised me when I was in Science and Non-duality (SAND) 2017 conference in San Jose, California. I witnessed a very famous spiritual guru answering the question about how to handle the trauma of the past.

He responded with the sentence, "You close the closet of past," and my opposition to or debating on this statement was never welcomed. I also did not feel the urge to argue more so I shut my mouth and listened to him that we are talking about very different types of consciousness. Anyhow, that was indeed a fantastic learning experience.

Neither our soul nor our learning ability is like a computer program. You can rewrite many times on the computer without consequences, according to our current and present needs. Therefore, there is no need at all to activate the past.

However, in-depth psychology has evidence that "the unconscious is not that it does not exist," as Freud said. It means that the unconscious exists and has its effects, although they are not observable.

According to Dr. Werner Meinhold's research, the analytical study above all in conscious hypnosis, clearly shows that past events supposedly forgotten long ago, can decisively influence lifestyle and cause very severe diseases. If those past events are deprogrammed or are removed forcefully without processing the psychodynamics, then the danger of symptom shift (symptom apparently disappears and appears again after some time) occurs.

From my practical knowledge of 21 years with thousands of clients treating them for conditions such as anxiety to psychosis, I have experienced and lived through his research in more than 20000 cases. Working with past origins helped them live more "permanent peaceful solutions," which further reduced their inner conflicts. They start living their life in harmony and more in acceptance with themselves and their surroundings.

Research done on "bad memories suppression" from the past resulted in blocking present-day memory formation. It means that it can lead people to have difficulties with their everyday memories of ordinary events. The study supports current approaches to tackling PTSD, which advises against suppressing recollections.

Psychoanalysis with conscious hypnosis does not reactivate a past of little importance. However, it makes aware of the old ballasts of life history present in its effects. It also opens up the possibility of treating them, freeing themselves from them through their conscious integration.

Who is responsible for my disease?

Nearly every human being tries to make another person feel responsible for his suffering one way or another. During hard times he went through pain because someone did something to cause it, and now he has to live with it for the rest of his life. This individual can be anybody. It can be his mom who rejected him after giving birth or his father, who deserted him. It can be a wife, a friend, or a son or a daughter, a relative, or even a stranger who has acted upon his life. He has no escape, and that event or series of events will affect him for the rest of his life.

He might surrender to the circumstances. When he feels hopeless to continue his life, he will take it as a lesson and devote his life to helping others. Either way, the objective of his life is not the same as it had been otherwise.

I saw a Tony Robbins documentary "I am not your Guru" on Netflix. I could not control my therapeutic assessment training from surfacing as I watched the show, so I tried to understand it at a deeper level. I observed some hidden triggers in his statements about his childhood relationship with his mother and how helping others became a kind of addiction. There can be a hidden connection between these two if we can tap into his unconscious and work through it.

The question that arises is this:" would he like to keep on working with the same passion and in the same field after those parts are uncovered, processed, and understood? Maybe, now there is no anxiety left pushing him unconsciously to help others.

Luis Miguel, a famous Mexican singer, likewise had a complicated childhood relationship with his parents. Although he achieved world fame and fortune as a singer, he suffered from depression. He was briefly admitted to a hospital in 2010 in Los Angeles. The cause of hospitalization remains a secret. Does he feel that his parents are responsible for his mental health issues? I cannot verify this until and unless I tap into his unconscious mind. However, I am more than confident that there is a pang of intense guilt or resentment hidden somewhere in his covert mind. I can name many of these examples and it may take years to write down all these cases. Nevertheless, it has given me an idea to write a book about some celebrities who felt that they were unconsciously driven to do one thing in their life, but perhaps they wanted to do to be something else.

We should never forget who we are. Before being anyone, whether a wealthy, famous, and adored superstar, or a poor, insignificant unknown from nowhere. Beneath all and above all, we are always going to remain human first. You cannot escape the essential nature of being a human, no matter how hard you try.

Every human being needs to connect with his inner self if he wants to live a harmonious and peaceful life. It also creates wonders when it comes to mental, physical, or spiritual health. Modern meditations and other mindfulness techniques can be helpful up to a certain point. However, they are not enough to fully explore and completely live the life of a "forever balanced and complete human being" until and unless you make your unconscious conscious.

The healing methods or techniques connected to work on the inner self has a much higher successful rate than the others. If you add conscious hypnosis to it, such as "Integrative therapy of in-depth Psychology" by Dr. Werner Meinhold. It can transform your life in a way you can't imagine. It has changed mine and thousands of others.

This therapeutic process helped me to control my life by exploring the possibility of not living anymore as a victim or blaming others. It provided the necessary tools and awareness to bring my center back. I accepted the responsibility of the events that occurred in my life with the lesson that I am — and no one else is — the creator of my life's experiences. Then moving onwards, I have applied the same pathway to guide others. They understood the importance of connecting with their inner-self. They found hidden answers for long-awaited questions appearing in their life as anxiety, depression, fears, suffering or other mental or physical disorders.

The healing methods of in-depth psychology aspire to discover and process causal connections in the history of life. From time to time, it arrives at an erroneous assumption that while finding a reason, a person who caused it also appears. Now we have 'someone blameworthy.'

Am I to blame for my illness or my parents are? Most of my clients often ask this question. Many parents have already received several reproaches and have transformed those reproaches against them.

Meinhold invites us to be mindful of the question by allowing us to look at the problem from a 'guilt' point of view. We have to differentiate among guilt from a legal point of view, ideas of moral guilt and psychoanalytic treatment with the questions regarding guilt.

The court or legal system hypothesizes that awareness of having done something wrong is sufficient to be proclaimed as being guilty. Parents proceed without knowing psychoanalytic understandings, and even they are convinced that this is the best for their child. However, they will give him a neurotic education from a psychoanalytic point of view. With this, they show the way, more or less consciously, to the norms inherited from their parents or the standards or rules set by society. The original guilt must return through grandparents and great grandparents to Adam and Eve.

People also tend to search for guilt concerning their behaviour. The responsible causes of early general childhood experiences have no apprehension of the connections that occur with subsequent developments or the possibility of totally different and intelligent behaviour.

The idea of moral guilt depends mainly on the social order, which serves the base for the conception of the world. What is rewarded in one country can be condemned in another. That is why it is indispensable for psychoanalytic work to investigate the psychic connections. Knowing the other side of rules and clear customs, which often can be neurotic and considering this social order as a reference system, but not as a scale of absolute value.

Therefore, the therapist should not play the role of a judge, priest in overseeing ideological or religious commandments or suggest to the patient his ideas and values. Preferably, he should accept the patient without conditions and as he is. This way, he promotes the growth and development through the therapeutic process, and the client by himself experiences an ethical and responsible vision of himself. It would be more difficult for him to understand and accept his life's story without his idea of his spiritual sense in many cases.

The therapeutic process does not have the task of blaming or forgiving. It helps to open up an understanding with one's respective connections and integrates the experiences that have so far been rejected in the history of life.

With this, the base for a conscious life with love, freedom and responsibility can be created, and bid a permanent goodbye to numerous physical, mental, or spiritual disorders.

"Your shadow is a confirmation that
you are in front of the sunshine."

"Since the moment I have deciphered pain,
love surrounds me everywhere."

Atul Mehra

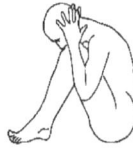

Chapter 8
What is Symptom?

A symptom can be a physical or mental characteristic that indicates ill health or disease. It can be a sign of an undesirable situation that does not allow one to live an everyday normal life.

According to Wiktionary, the word symptom comes from the Ancient Greek *sumptoma*, which is a happening, an accident or a symptom of a disease. It is from the stem of *sumpipto*, meaning I befall, which is "sum," and "pipto" meaning I fall.

I love this explanation of symptoms, especially the Greek word *sum* meaning together. It implies a message which states *please do not ignore me as I am a part of you, and we need to resolve it together to become one or whole.* A person creates the symptoms by himself, unconsciously conscious; he had some bad experiences in the past. They are presented as symptoms in his present life because nobody buys his disease from another person.

The presence of a symptom is something logical. Our body is wise enough to find and create the perfect symptom. It is the opposite of me, and it helps me to recognize myself. The opposite is essential in our life. The opposite brings balance because balance comes from extremities. For example, the day is opposite to the night and vice-versa, and they sustain the continuation of life. Complete all-time darkness or night on the planet will end life, and so would the total light or day forever. Having said that, symptoms of a disease is the exact opposite of health. It is as if the natural course of health has been interrupted by illness. The natural flow of life's river is filled with obstacles. Sometimes this river overflows while continuing its pathway, and the water floods into the surrounding regions. Can we imagine the presence of disease in our life as an overflowing river that is causing other areas to be also affected?

Who creates the symptom? The patient himself does; most of the therapeutic processes find answers to why the symptom exists and work only with one part of the brain, but they should never be relieving the symptom. However, the therapist should act as a counsellor or a lawyer representing the patient's personality that is creating the symptoms. Instead of trying to answer why, therapy ought to focus on the "what for" or what the patient is trying to express through his symptoms.

"Why" and "What for" look very similar but they are not. They have a significant difference when it comes to rethinking your life and setting your goals. The mental processes involved are the opposite.

When you ask 'why", your mind goes back to the past and brings up rational causes that led you to a circumstance or a particular situation. It takes you to a path of justifications, which can be historical or conditional.

For example, if I ask you, "why are you alive?", you might respond with "what" and a smile, but your mind might come up with the answer *because of my parents, they got married and I took birth...*

"Why do you work?" Because I have to earn money so I could eat, pay the rent and bills, and other expenses. You can also say that you can't afford to be out of a job or maybe you enjoy working.

Now let's discuss the other question. When I ask you "what for," then your awareness looks to the future, awakening the true meaning of what you do and what drives you to do what you do from the heart. It activates the emotional brain, which is the right hemisphere, creativity, imagination and sleep. It takes you to the hidden patterns working underneath for what you do.

Example: What for you are alive? You decide to love, to grow, to learn, to give, to evolve, to enjoy and to succeed.

What for do you work? To learn, do my best, contribute to a team or to the community, achieve goals, live what makes you feel passionate about something.

The answer "why" points to the causes, often external, that bring you to this moment. "What for" places you in a creative space that calls for a purpose and reason for being.

The "why" is easy to answer. Just look back and find the causes for working. The "why" may lack meaning and emotion.

The "what for" puts you in a context of meaning, purpose, and infinite possibilities. It is the fuel that makes you go, what charges you to get up in the morning and live your life with consciousness, enthusiasm and passion.

Asking yourself "why" satisfies your mind and "what for" fills your heart.

Have you been wondering lately "what for" are you doing what you are doing?

Have you decided "what for" you want what you want?

Although many people do not understand at the beginning when I ask them, "what for?" They repeat "why?" and I say again, "No, what for?" and I explain, which opens up the possibilities to understand a deeper meaning. I hope I have provided clarity so please do let me know if you still have any questions, please, and if so, then "what for"? LOL

The questions remain: why does the symptom exists and how can we deal with it and heal from it? Is it possible to know its origins? Can we process it, understand it, and integrate it back as part of natural living that enables one to live a "sum" of life as a whole?

There are hundreds of different types of therapeutic approaches to treat a client, but we can divide them into three main types. They can be

Emotional mind therapy, Rational (logical-analytical) mind therapy, and Integrative or holistic therapy.

One of the remarkable therapeutic approaches is Emotionally Focused Therapy (EFT). According to an article at goodtherapy.com, some psychological issues, such as panic or impulse control, can be described as disproportionate responses to one's subjective reality. These parts of experience might include thoughts, feelings, or bodily sensations. EFT helps people be more responsive to their inner experience. Due to this, it is generally not recommended in the treatment of these issues.

EFT requires people to be open and honest. It helps people develop a compassionate stance toward their own emotional experience. Nevertheless, this treatment is generally not meant for those who may deliberately deceive or manipulate the therapist.

EFT is a type of therapy aimed at improving a person's overall functioning. It does not address specific symptoms. So, it may not be as useful for people seeking treatment to reduce a particular mental health symptom.

The other drawback of this kind of therapeutic process can be for the client; it is as if one were opening a Pandora's box. It can be excruciating and quite exhausting, re-living past traumatic experiences. It may well mean that the client will indeed feel worse before the benefits begin to manifest. It is sometimes challenging to have to work with the premise that one cannot go forward until they have gone back.

I have had clients who used therapeutic approaches to work on their emotions. The main objective was to handle emotional issues and go back to a normotic healthy life as quickly as possible. Accessing and working directly with those memories resulted in a lot of pain, suffering, and in some cases, suicidal thoughts.

Rational mind therapeutic approaches work with the logical, analytical mind and bring faster results. Coping techniques, such as Cognitive Behaviour Therapy (CBT), help us to take fast control over stressful circumstances.

A panic attack situation can come under control through a particular visualization, meditation and other indirect methods. We can consider all of them as a part of the behaviour therapy.

Behaviour therapy or behaviour psychology treat mental health disorders. It identifies and helps change self-destructive or unhealthy behaviours. The principles of behaviourism tend to look at specific, learned behaviour and how the environment influences those behaviours.

Some action-based therapies focus on current problems and how to change them. These therapies are CBT, Applied Behaviour Analysis (ABA), Role Playing, Desensitization and other relaxation techniques. All these techniques indirectly help the client to cope with his mental disorder and create control over the current situation. He is encouraged to repeat the same process every time he faces the same problem. I have worked with many clients who before coming to me took part in behaviour therapy techniques for a panic attack. They worked with coping techniques that included deep breathing, self-talk, and identifying situations that they often avoided and gradually worked with situations that caused fear. Those techniques helped them to control the circumstances up to a certain extent, and occasionally they helped in some situations and at other times not at all. The consistent use of coping techniques to deal with a panic attack created a vicious circle. It resulted in a lot of confusion, inner-struggle and exhaustion. Instead of going to the root cause or to the *seed* of the problem, they went around in circles and ultimately learned to live with it or, in some cases, took medications as means of dealing with their feelings.

I am not at all against practicing behaviour therapy as they can be of great help and value to many people. I always suggest working on the origins of the symptom in order to get a kind of permanent solution or longer-lasting results.

What exactly happens in behaviour therapy? It reprograms the client's behaviour according to upbringing or Superego. According to Freud, the Superego incorporates the values and morals of society learned from one's parents, society, culture, religion, education, and environment. It can also include the period from the mother's womb to the first five years of age.

The symptoms disappear but the client goes back to the state before the symptoms. On the other end, a therapist uses his technique and applies his normotic ideas to the client, generally making the symptoms disappear and returning to the state before the symptoms. Can we call it a pathological regression back to square one?

Both processes can be considered as illogical because they go back to the state before the symptom. It can also lead to the great danger of relocation of symptoms or symptoms shift (explained in the next paragraphs with more details). Thus, the individuality and spirituality of the client are not respected because he has to find by himself his solutions while integrating the unrecognized part of his "self" and energies, which are previously hiding beneath his symptoms. Integrative in-depth psychology therapy (THIPP) works with the same principle and requires the client's conscious collaboration.

THIPP is a holistic and integrative therapeutic approach that has blended elements from different methods and has a proven record of a much higher success rate. Integrative therapy of depth psychology was born in Germany between 1971 and 1997. It remained in the process of continuous development since then, thanks to the theoretical contribution of students and colleagues and practical application in patients. This therapy was developed and structured by Dr. Werner J. Meinhold.

THIPP is a new holistic therapeutic approach that is simultaneously highly specific, connecting human, social and natural sciences with depth psychology, Gestalt consciousness or the form, hypnotic awareness.

The principles of this therapy can be applied in all areas of daily life and used as therapy, offering real help for all kinds of disturbances and diseases. It helps each individual by strengthening the Self in this world so he can express his true nature.

In this therapeutic process, we unbutton the buttons placed in the wrong buttonholes of the shirt from bottom to top. Imagine going down to the depths of the dangerous hidden basement of the psyche through a ladder, slowly and carefully, one step at a time.

In the basement of the psyche, the repressed and isolated parts of the Self are hidden, including all the existential anxieties. These existential anxieties are inaccessible in the conscious adult mind. This is because they are under the custody of the censuring unconscious.

According to Meinhold, accessing these parts too quickly can cause an inundation of unconscious with severe trauma for the client, which can lead to them leaving the therapeutic process, create psychosis or attempt suicide.

The famous German poet Goethe used the metaphor of shirt buttons to describe this process. If you make a mistake with the first button of the shirt by putting in the wrong buttonhole, then the first buttonhole remains empty. You keep on buttoning the remaining buttons in incorrect buttonholes. The same thing happens with a deficit development of the first phase of life, which occurs intra-uterine or during pregnancy, and keeps occurring with the rest of the stages of life, each getting affected by the previous one. Usually, one does not detect the error until arriving at the last buttonhole and realizing that a button is leftover, but the buttonholes have run out.

In the same way, the symptoms that occur are often only visible above the conscious or surface level. We need to work at the earliest stages of life's story until we reach the conditions of origin.

Taking into account the law of the first button the client often presents superficial symptoms, which are simply a mask for more profound problems.

A holistic therapeutic approach, such as THIPP, can work through these masks and make other layers of symptoms visible beneath them. Once the nucleus of the disorder becomes evident, we can easily find its base in the intrauterine life.

Every therapeutic process, whether with drugs or suggestions when used against symptoms, carries the risk that symptoms come from a deeper physical or psychological level. If such symptoms disappear, there is an illusion that the disturbance is over. However, if it has its origin on a deeper level, it has to find other forms of expression, which are usually more severe than the first. This process is called *Relocation of symptoms or Symptoms shift* and was discovered by Dr. Reckweg at the physical level. Dr. Werner Meinhold has described its validity for the psychic level and the connections between both levels.

The *Symptom Shift* can last for months to years and appears again different than the original problem. If another anti-symptomatic treatment occurs, it produces the next transfer of symptoms, until it reaches complete deterioration. The symptoms can shift from the physical level to the mental level and vice versa. Here is an example of symptoms shift on the physical level from mild to severe.

Humoral Phases (liquid Level)

1. Excretion (e.g., Heavy sweating)

2. Reaction (e.g., Skin inflammation).

3. Disposition in body fluids (e.g., A latent poisoning)

Biological Cut (division between humoral and cellular level)

Cellular stages (at the structural level)

1. Impregnation (e.g., Osteoarthritis)

2. Degeneration (e.g., Sclerosis)

3. Neoplasm (e.g., Cancer)

Mental stages, according to Meinhold, are:

1. Neurotic Level (Mental level)

2. Strong feelings (e.g., Anger)

3. Extreme feelings (e.g., Unbearable fears)

4. Embedded Conflicts (e.g., a transfer to the unconscious fear)

Borderline (division between the neurological level and psychotic level) Psychotic phases (at the level of the person)

1. Fixation (e.g., Addictions and compulsions).

2. Depression (e.g., Cyclothymia)

3. Psychosis (e.g., Paranoia, Schizophrenia, hearing voices etc.)

Symptoms can jump from the physical level to the mental level and vice versa. In the THIPP approach developed by Werner Meinhold, the individual travels through the *causal* road returning to previous states up to the healing. A simple example of this is when a person holding on to anger may begin to sweat heavily. The task is to create harmony between different levels, i.e., physical, mental and beyond, to integrate all parts of the personality of a patient to become one.

Any symptom and its origins are in our mind and their solution too. An induced relaxation state can help access those parts and, through a "wider framing process," can make the symptom go away.

Our mind records every second of experiences lived by us throughout our life. The total capacity of the brain is 10 to the power of 80. It is the same as the approximate quantity of atoms in the universe. It means that we can easily record the experiences of every second of 1000 years! The part we know as the conscious or logical-analytical mind is approximately 0.0000000001% of the total capacity.

Our life experiences from sperm consciousness until this present moment are stored in our memory bank. They can be accessed easily under a conscious relaxation state as long as there is no unconscious resistance.

Experiences lived by us in the mother's womb or early childhood cannot be explained or rationalized. That is because as a child we did not possess the analytical skills of an adult.

A special incident took place in the past that impacted a client's life. It has been recorded in the foreground of his memory, which is also the subconscious memory. He has limited access to that memory, more like a brief glimpse of a fact that something terrible happened. However, he consciously cannot access the whole memory of it, and this indirectly affects his present life. Thus, he cannot find any connection between the incident and his present situation.

These unpleasant experiences are filtered through one's perception of the event and will only access select memories that resonate with his neurotic beliefs. We can regard memory as a picture in a tiny frame that is so small that we cannot see all the smaller details that make up the complete picture.

In order to magnify the picture, we need to broaden the frame. We can facilitate a broader view of the original event without therapeutic falsification of life history. Then the client, by himself, can recognize those previously repressed parts by the neurotic limits of his perception and integrate the image in his life's story. In a nutshell, the idea is to make that client fully visible, that which has been invisible his entire life.

The appropriate method to amplify the framework in other cases can be done by connecting with the person through telepathy and, at the same time, recognizing the deep levels of transference and countertransference of the event in question.

https://blog.oup.com/2016/04/mother-teresa-depression/

"Every physical disease or a mental disorder is an unrecognized, unspoken, unconscious part of the self."

Atul Mehra

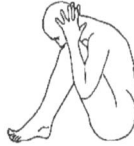

Chapter 9
The Need for Disease

" Behave yourself, or I will give you my cancer!" How ludicrous and unbelievable this sentence would sound even if we say it once. We all want to live a healthy life. How exactly do we define health? You might argue that being healthy means living free from illness, injury, or pain. Would you consider a person to be healthy if he had neither smoked nor drank a day in his life, followed rigorous healthy eating habits, and took great care of his health in all possible ways, and yet died at the age of 40 from a heart attack? Looking at these factors raises questions about the definition of health, we focus our attention on exploring the true meaning of health.

Can life be planned rationally and include space for disease? No one consciously sets out to acquire diabetes at the age of 15, multiple sclerosis at a young age of 25, cancer at age 30, or die at 32 years of age. Yet, we know of loved ones or friends who have been affected by these and other serious illnesses resulting in death at an early age. Who or what is responsible for this situation? Is it me, the society or somebody else, who is responsible? People spend their entire lives blaming others and get an erroneous belief that leads them to ask, "Who is responsible for my disease?"

The research on depth psychology has proven that the intrauterine life, development of early childhood stages and early life experiences play a significant role in adult life. Every mental or physical disorder can be a consequence of an unconscious defective impregnation of one or more of these growth periods. The individual himself creates it.

Realizing that we create our disease and knowing the origin requires us to go to a deeper level. It is the key that unlocks the mysteries of disease creation and provides us with hopeful pathways to restore our health and wellbeing. Whether it is cancer, diabetes, anxiety or any other physical or mental disorder, it is the individual himself who creates it at an unconscious level.

The presence of disease in one's life is always a misfortune. Today I would like to share something that rests outside of the traditional health system box. I am tired of getting a line about the different definitions of health conditions. The disease is unkind, and I support this idea; in other words, when you are sick, it is essential to go to the doctor for medical assessment and treatment. I urge that once the treatment of the symptoms begins, and the person feels relief, it is a prime opportunity to recognize that this work has just started and continues to go deeper to understand the disease process. That is where I want to share something that some of you may not willingly take. However, I will give it my best effort to help you understand health and disease from an out-of-the-box perspective. That will set you free from the confines within which you had been viewing them.

The origin of a disease can begin at the stage of a sperm consciousness. When induced into a consciously relaxed state, a person can access his unconscious brain and discover whether he was accepted as a baby. It becomes the seed for his future life and for attracting all his life experiences accordingly. Those first emotional experiences impact and indirectly control our lives all the time -- 24/7 and 365 days of the year. We may imagine that we live a conscious life, but in reality, that percentage is deficient, perhaps 5% or less. Amazingly, the consciousness of life begins before sperm consciousness, but that is a different story that I will share some other time. My intention here is to explain my research and findings based on scientific evidence that I gathered about the origins of human life and wellness in its physical form.

Life begins from a single cell consciousness in the mother's womb, and, after passing through millions of processes, it reaches a totality of the form to become ONE or a whole being. From that very second to all the future hours of "now as today," these procedures require the best possible unconditional growth of the self. Continuous obstacles, repressions or going against those operations can create future mental or physical illnesses.

97% of all people do not know that our body possesses the capacity to heal itself from any disease. We can create illness and we can heal it too. We are not mindful of our inner strength. We depend so much upon external resources and physical aspects of being a human to fight against diseases and get quick relief from symptoms. We go back to the state before the symptoms began, continue the same path as before when we received warning signs or just produce entirely different symptoms, and keep on cycling through the creation and disappearance of symptoms for the rest of our lives.

I am not stating the use of medicines are useless, but rather that while using the medication, it is also of utter importance to integrate the working and accessing of the unconscious mind to find where the seeds of illness lie.

I will illustrate an example: Bruce Lee, one of the most energetic people in the world, yet he died at 32 years of age. It is widely believed that he died of cerebral edema; there are still many rumours circulating about his untimely death. Was he unable to face his underlying fears created during his childhood or was it something else? We will never know the real truth unless we explore the depths of unconsciousness and begin to understand the malignant energy lurking beneath any disease.

Can a heart attack, stroke or fatal accident be an unconscious pattern of committing suicide? We will not know until we are willing to see how our unconscious mind works and the connections working within it.

You may be surprised to find out that although Mother Teresa sacrificed her life for the betterment of humanity, she suffered from periodic depression, a chronic form of the emotional darkness created by her on an unconscious level. Does it mean by serving others the path she took was nothing but to fill a dark void within her that formed in her childhood? All these questions remain a mystery and challenge us to set about shifting our perspective. They guide us to research the patterns that are related to our unconscious mind to create a need for the disease.

The other invisible example of society's recommendation is to have fame and wealth. Our whole life we are surrounded by this. It was implanted in our subconscious since we are conceived or maybe even before. I would also like to add the example of famous actor Robin Williams. His extraordinary work not only left a significant influence on my heart but also on that of millions of people. He had everything, wealth, fame, many partners, and all other "luxuries of life" and yet he was driven to commit suicide. Why? What went wrong in his life?

The research again points at a person's unconscious hidden patterns at work. I am confident that now that we are nearing the end of this book, you are becoming aware of this important topic. Many questions have their answers, and new problems and curiosities about life have begun appearing on the surface. The same sensations and satisfaction I started feeling when I embark on discovering the secrets hidden in the depth of unconsciousness. Since then, my life has completely transformed. I live my life with more awareness, and my analytical brain works more in harmony with my emotional brain. Life makes more sense to me than before.

Every moment I have lived so far was a present moment at some time in my life. Every moment created a memory, an experience, my past or my life's story. Whatever went on at that time was the "best that happened" for that moment. However, my limited awareness of that moment memorized and recorded it as a bad malignant experience. Now it affects my present life because everything is "present" in the subconscious mind. There is no past or future, although I can rationalize it from an analytical point of view.

All these experiences are likewise a part of self or me. They run and interpret an essential role in my life. They are misunderstood because of the lack of complete awareness to understand them altogether. They need their expression so that they can be recognized and get their integration to become one. I name it "The Misunderstood Self or even better The Unspoken Self." It means that anxiety, depression, or disease is an unconscious expression of self. Your body is straining to say something to you, which you ignored in your life story, somehow knowing or unknowingly.

The idea is to make the unconscious conscious to understand the malignant energies working underneath the repetitive patterns causing the symptoms. Even Carl Jung said, "Until you make the unconscious conscious, it will direct your life, and you will call it fate." Even historic teachings, whether scientific, religious, self-help or spiritual all try to connect with self-awareness.

As I have mentioned before, a disease's origin can begin at the stage of Sperm consciousness or even earlier. During my 23 years of research, I found that everything starts in the mother's womb. In my published book *The Unseen Wisdom of the Unborn*, I explained how a mother's thoughts impact her baby's formation. However, there is no such thing as a bad mother; without her, we would not be here today.

We need to explore the depths of the unconscious and find new answers to understand the basic need for a disease. Disease is not the enemy; it is an opportunity to restore health and balance in your body, mind, and spirit. It is the missing piece of the puzzle that looks for its acceptance and helps to process the complete understanding of the event, which once created trauma in your life span.

Disease is a question and health is the answer. Both health and illness are components of the same soul. The soul of illness is the same as the soul of health. They have fallen apart, but at present, they are seeking a union to become one, which is also the Greek word "Sum."

Everybody creates an experience for a reason. If I withdraw pain or illness without understanding the process of creation or the lesson hidden underneath, then the opportunity for growth is lost, and each subsequent lesson gets tougher.

Answers and solutions lie within us. Solutions are created before problems, and problems are the bridge to solutions. Solutions are waiting to be discovered. All solutions lie within us as do all the problems. The only individual who can heal you is you because you created the disease, and its solution also lies within you.

People fear diseases, and as a human being it is natural to feel afraid because the awareness of fear makes us more human. However, we cannot escape from being sick, or God forbidding, sometimes even a terminal disease. Having said that, it becomes of utmost importance to the process to understand and integrate so that suffering can be minimized, and we head back towards better health.

The holistic way to look at the process of cancer can be considered not a way to die, but maybe, the last opportunity to live. It is a small, thin thread onto which the person is hanging. It can turn back if the person is willing to accept, understand and learn from it before it is too late.

In my experience, I have found out that every disease is psychosomatic. It implies a physical illness caused or aggravated by a mental factor such as internal conflict or stress. It means that first the symptoms appear in mind and then they manifest in the body. It is your mind, the conscious and the unconscious, looking for opportunities to work together as one human mind — the Self or I.

In that respect is the physiology of disease. There is a psychology of disease, and there is a spirituality of disease.

There is a need to integrate the spiritual part of the self. I do not mean to state that our spiritual self relates to religion or anything like that; instead, I refer to the essence of being human on all levels, whether during a time when we are healthy and when we are not healthy. Spirituality means accepting your role in every experience you bring into your life and accepting that you are the creator of your life. You equally accept responsibility for any experience with another human being, whether good or bad. A spiritual person experiences every moment of his life that we are all One, and consciously attempts to honour this Oneness as whole or togetherness.

Every mental or physical disorder can result from an unconscious defective interpretation of one or more of these growth periods and is; therefore, the person creates himself. We cannot access the experiences lived in the past with our present-day memory, and those hidden parts are the decision-makers in everyday life. They are controlling our every action and thought based on what we learnt in early childhood. If any part of the personality is not integrated in a healthy and understanding manner, then your body expresses it through disease. It may be a healthy expression of a point of view, but we call it a pathology or a disease when we study it from a rational point of view. It is what I regard as "the need for the disease."

When you are sick, you go to the doctor for medical assessment and treatment. My recommendation would be that once the treatment of disappearing symptoms begins and the person feels relief, it is a prime opportunity to recognize that this work has just started and to continue to go to a deeper level to understand the process of disease.

The process of the disease takes off and ends with the recognition and integration of it. It commences with the self and ends with the self too. In other words, when self or I create the disease. I recognize, process, understand and integrate the illness, which I name Self-Recognition. I accept and learn from the experiences and lessons created by the disease as a part of the past; I call Self-Acceptance. I open up the possibilities to live my life in this very present moment or now and here (Space and time), which I call Self-Present. I use those experiences in the present life to live as a whole or complete, which I call Self-Consciousness. It might not make sense, but "Nothing makes sense, and everything makes sense too, you decide."

Behind every war, every crime, or every case of cancer, schizophrenia, anxiety, anger or any physical, mental, and spiritual disease, or a choice to live a life that is happy or sad, poor, or rich, helping others or not, there is only one singular thing that everyone is looking for, and that is **acceptance**.

"Just for today, imagine your parents
smiling at you in your heart."

Atul Mehra

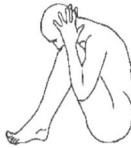

Chapter 10
Make Peace with your Mom and Dad in your Heart

In our modern world, people always give more importance to the mother than the father. It is perfectly true that the mother keeps the baby for 9 months in her womb, protects it and takes care of it the best possible way according to her circumstances. She may provide unconditional love, kindness, and protection, or the complete opposite, such as rejecting the baby because of its sex, abandoning it, having thoughts of aborting, or giving up the baby. In fact, she acts the best she can and there can be no better example of her love for you than you being here reading this book.

Some mothers go through very hard times during pregnancy and live through undesirable circumstances, which creates an impression on the unborn baby that he is unloved and is being rejected, although that may not be mother's feelings, emotions, desires or ideas, but the unborn reacts without understanding that those feelings are not associated with him because he does not have an intellectual capacity of an adult to process and understand it. The mother feels it so, he feels it too and that creates a kind of rejection towards mother and life goes around filling the gap for his unconscious quest for mother's love by doing something good or bad, the essential desire to feel loved or accepted.

Unconsciously, although father presence is equally important, but nevertheless it is believed that the world can go ahead without a father but not without a mother. It is a faulty concept. The unconscious psyche, whether an unborn baby, a child, an adult, or a senior citizen, all equally yearn for father's love, no matter what.

Although you are a unique person the cellular information or the DNA in you is part of your father and part of your mother. Both the sperm and the ovum joined together to create you. It means that a part in you belongs to your father and another part belongs to your mother. If you have issues with your father or mother the corresponding parts will experience those issues too, and it will be manifested into a physical or mental illness.

My therapeutic experience has taught me that illnesses can be developed in cases where we do not get along with our parents. Instead, I would say all infirmities or strengths in life move around the relationship with the parents. If you hold a good relationship with your parents, you are likely to feel more satisfied in your life. Bad relationship with your parents can lead to mental, physical, and spiritual pain.

Every client I have ever seen in my life, no matter what physical, mental or spiritual discordance they had, whether it was a mental disorder such as anxiety, depression, psychosis, sadness, dissatisfaction, loneliness, suicidal thoughts, or a physical ailment such as cancer, asthma, chronic pain, or addiction, whenever I start working and going to the deepest roots of their present problems, connections with Mom and Dad start to appear. Those subtle connections were eye-opening and surprising for my clients as they never thought they would one day discover their parents as the origin of their present problems. However, later in therapy they find with relief that their parents were never the origin of their problems, but rather it was their interpretations of those moments at their unconscious level that gave rise to the conditions causing the illness. Once this was made visible, they were accepted, processed, understood, and integrated and given a clear pathway to health, satisfying relationships, and even improved financial opportunities.

Parents play a very significant role in our lives. They did what they could at that time and that was the best they could do. Dwelling on a belief that one's mom could have done better or one's father should have been that way is just a waste of time and is not going to resolve anything in your life; instead, it creates more anxiety which leads to loneliness and isolation and destroys the joys of present moments that can be experienced in a more fulsome and meaningful way.

You cannot change the story of your life. You cannot spend your life wishing that your father was a great king and your mother a queen (may be in some cases, but they must have their own issues too, and I don't want to mention it, but you understand what I am referring to) and they loved you unconditionally. What you have lived so far that has only been the pathway to get where you are now. It attaches a great importance to the fact that you have to accept the account of your life and make peace with it. The pathway you have found to get here in your present life was the only solution and others were just not possible. You have to take them as they are and start analyzing how to start living your life from now on. Getting to make peace with mom, dad, and everyone, including yourself is key in living life more in harmony physically, mentally, and spiritually.

The mind here is to make peace with mom and dad, no matter what. If it is physically possible to do that and they are receptive to it, then I would strongly recommend doing that and if you think you have resistance then you can go for therapeutic help to resolve the unconscious resistance and make it happen. In case that is not possible, then at least you should establish peace in your heart by opening it and allowing yourself to look at them from the point of view of love and compassion. Bringing awareness that they are also human being like you, and they must have their own reasons to be as they are — maybe it was a learned behaviour from their parents, or circumstances in life pushed them into uncontrollable situations. Looking at the things from their point of view will serve you to understand their pain and limitations and this is the only way to heal yourself and make peace with people around you. The bad relationship with your parents in your subconscious mind can also indirectly affect your relationship with your children or spouse.

Many of your issues with your parents can be characterized as examples of unconscious hooks. I can explain it with a real example. A young client of mine experienced severe breathing problems. This could have been fatal during those times that his breathing was restricted, and every time he suffered through those episodes, his mother felt it even though she was far away from him working out of the house. She called the maid every time she felt it who confirmed back as saying that he was indeed going through labored breathing. The mother explained that she used to have that gut feeling that something bad is happening to her son, and when she called him to talk to him, he subsequently calmed down just listening to her reassuring voice. During his sessions, the son explored that he felt a kind of a need to connect with his mother and the only way he found that she responded quickly was to unconsciously create a situation with a severe breathing problem. Once resolved, his breathing issues disappeared miraculously.

Illustrated by the example above, we can understand how we relate to the person we love, and we find good or bad ways to connect with them or to be with them. I have someone really close who says, "I reject my father and he rejects me" and I respond," you are connecting with your father through rejection, which is common, but underneath, love is waiting to be manifested."

The transference and countertransference in above example explain that the event is taking place on an unconscious level. We don't know who the sender is and who the receiver is, or who the judge is and who the victim is, as it is all happens reciprocally. The mother senses that something is wrong with my son, and he feels that mother is anxious when he is not breathing well. They link up with each other, unconsciously, simultaneously and beyond time and limit.

I am certain that if you begin with this awareness, you will see many such examples around you and in your life. One of the great examples can be when Carrie Fisher, who is known for playing Princess Leia in the Star Wars movies, died of a sudden cardiac arrest. Her mother, Debbie Reynolds, the famous American actress, singer, and businesswoman, also suffered a severe stroke the following day and died. According to her, she wanted to be with her daughter, and she did not desire to leave her daughter alone. She had been seriously moved by her daughter's death and her grief was partially responsible for her stroke.

Human existence is founded on love. Love surrounds us in different forms and if it does not gain its true significance, it transforms into hate, fear, separation, and/or pain. It can further transmute into mental or physical pain and lead to terminal mental or physical diseases.

Once you have found peace with your parents, you will be surprised how things start to change in your life. The sense of understanding towards your parents will bring rewards in its own way in every area of your life and you will feel more connected internally than before. I could construct a list of million benefits of making peace with your parents but rather I encourage you to experience it on your own.

From the bottom of my heart and with honesty I recommend this to you.

The clock is ticking away, and every precious moment is coming off. Allow yourself to consider the idea to get on better with your parents. Then, go to your parents and make peace with them in your heart and continue making peace with each and every person you come across and then write to me about your experience. If you try and you do not feel any better, then it means that more work is needed on an unconscious level, and I will make it happen with a few sessions at my clinic. How does that sound?

"Life is not about balance.
It is about living.

The balance naturally comes when
you start living your own life."

Atul Mehra

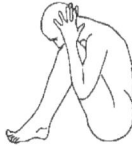

Chapter 11
If You Create your Disease,
then You can Heal it too

Have you ever wondered why in life we have easily learned and experienced creating an illness, but eradicating it from our lives has been like moving a mountain? Imagine that in one instant life is running smoothly and everything is coming up roses for you, and then suddenly in the next instant something unforetold happens -- you discover that you have a major (or even a minor) health issue. You feel severe anxiety and a plethora of other emotions relating to your diagnosis which begin to dominate your life. A variety of worrisome thoughts related to how problematic your life will become begin to take up valuable space in your mind. It gets to a point where it morphs into something huge and becomes impossible to handle.

As soon as something goes wrong, God forbid, you immediately begin to live your life as though it were missing something big. This is the "missing tile syndrome" which takes a prominent role in your life, and you begin to live vicariously through it. I remember when I started losing my hair at an early age. I always looked for people with less hair in a social gathering to make myself feel better. It was a source of shame for me and the reason for being teased during my adolescence. I suffered a great deal of shame and pain and tried different hairstyles to cover the growing baldness. I wasted a lot of time, money and efforts and sometimes felt a grudge against my parents and grandparents because they were bald. In those moments, I almost forgot that I had other qualities that could easily overcome my minor drawback. One of the biggest challenges was when anybody looked at me, their eyes immediately went to my growing baldness, and I could glimpse a glimmer of pity in their eyes.

Bit by bit, when I started accepting myself, I used the strategy of using humour as a turning point while socializing to break the ice by joking about my increased baldness, referring it to as a half or ascending moon. People laughed and shared, and since then, nobody has looked at me with the same eyes before. I realized then on a much deeper level how I attract what I feel.

One day I fully accepted my baldness and decided to shave my head to make it a full moon (LOL), and since then, I have received many compliments that I have a perfectly shaped head for being bald. I figured out that my external world changes if my internal world changes. I have never been so proud of my success in accepting myself as a whole person who flows with the natural rhythm of life. All this time, my anxiety and suffering have been trying to tell me what I had not been doing. Does this make any sense to you?

The "missing tile syndrome" refers to irregularities and flaws. Imagine a patchwork of fifty beautiful tiles together, and one of them is missing. You will appreciate and enjoy the patchwork, but if asked your opinion, most of the time, your first question will be about the missing tile. What happened to it? Did it fall from the wall, or was it somehow missed amongst the rest? You might say to yourself, "Such a beautiful patchwork, but if that missing tile were there, then things would have been different." Are you living your life with a missing tile syndrome?

Occasionally, everyone experiences setbacks and there is no escape from it. A person with an illness or a health challenge begins to live his life through that incompleteness and forgets that he has other parts that make up his healthy and active body. Is it possible to become mindful of our own missing tile syndrome and start living our lives differently?

The presence of any disease, illness, or any mental disorder can be related to our intrauterine life experiences and the first five years of our age. The language you learn is the language you speak. For instance, let us say the first language in your life was English and when you were learning it from your parents, you never challenged them about what they were teaching you or whether it was right or wrong. You grew up and developed the rationalization skills of a mature, analytical mind that could think, process, and speak English fluently even though you could not remember how you learned it. Suppose today you happen to learn a new language such as Spanish. In that learning process, you will undoubtedly use your rational mind to explain certain words from various perspectives. You can also challenge the multiple meanings of a particular word from a rational standpoint, something you could not do when you were learning your first language at an early age.

At the same time, English becomes the root and reference to learn a new language.

Having said that, whatever you saw, learned, heard, imagined, felt, thought, or lived during the first five years of your age inclusive of intrauterine life became the root in which you would attract experiences for the rest of your life. Most likely, the first masculine image of a man in your life is that of your father. Likewise, the first feminine image of a woman in your life is that of your mother. Generally, your Mom or Dad are both present in your early life. However, if the son does not meet his father – either due to his death or abandonment -- he creates a telepathic connection with the father and takes on many or all his characteristics into him. You might have experienced or heard of instances where a son has never met his father, yet people who knew the father would claim, "although you never met your father, you are very similar to him." In case where the father has passed away, the son connects to a near father-like relative and transfers his characteristics on to himself.

These early childhood conditioning measures are in control – they are in the driver's seat. They influence our everyday thoughts, decisions, behaviours, and attitudes, as well as the possibilities to create choices and decisions that become very limited in everyday life. Almost every client I have had has realized that his previous lifestyle was wrong. However, before that discovery, he believed that they had perfect and complete acceptance of others' actions and behaviours, and that was perfectly normal. For example, my clients often learned that sharing and spending time with their children is a healthy way of loving them instead of going out to work and giving them material things such as computers, cars, or other such items. It is not a healthy way to love children because what they need most is to feel a close bond to their parents through sharing, spending time, and doing things together that makes them feel secure and loved. Parents raising young children have learn this pattern of behaviour from their own parents. It was a normotic pathological way to show their love to their children, resulting in rejection and painful relationships with their children. Making the unconscious conscious of their earliest intrauterine and childhood experiences helped to transform their relationship with their children into loving, respectful, and understanding relationships.

My own life experiences lead me to conclude that every disease or mental disorder is psychosomatic. It first appears in your psychic level and then later, if not resolved, shows up in the body (soma).

I remember once Dr. Meinhold talked about "Oncología del Idioma" in Spanish. It sounds strange to translate it directly into English as "Oncology of an idiom." It has a profound meaning and took me much time to understand what it meant after I worked with hundreds of clients. Oncology is the study of cancer. The word "Idioma" does not refer here to the English word "idiom," but it translates as the word "language" in English. It means the correct translation would be "Oncology of a language." He talked about research about the possibility that if someone were to find a proper word for its corresponding disease, then that disease disappears and integrates back into health.

For example, when you say, "I do not want to smoke," then your old brain rejects the words "don't want" and receives the message "I smoke." The old brain has its structure and processing mechanism, and it generates emotions and impulses accordingly. That is why decisions imposed by the rational mind (cerebral cortex or neocortex) have limitations when it comes to creating long-lasting benign results. Instead, it brings more struggle and dividedness in the long term. The basic need to become whole or complete can transform into a long-lasting, unsatisfied, painful emptiness. Consider this: I forgive you, but I do not forget you. Our old brain does not understand the new analytical language, and it rejects the negation, prefix, and suffix of the rational language as it has been described through an example above.

Our bodies can create disease and it has the same capacity to heal it too. My experience confirms that this healing capacity is hidden somewhere deep down in dark depths of our unconscious mind. We need to work within our deepest psychic level for healthy integration to occur.

We cannot rationalize it till we bring it up to our awareness, and then it becomes pliable in our rational sphere so it can be merged into a united whole. Many therapeutic techniques can help reach that awareness, but they have severe limitations to incorporate it back without guilt, feeling victim or something similar. These therapeutic methods generally work like one-way traffic to relieve and make symptoms disappear which only contribute to short-term results; this later causes a symptom shift or relocation of symptoms.

They do not make visible both sides of the situations, which I call Transferential Awareness, Acceptance, Understanding and Integration (TAAUI) and Counter-Transferential Awareness, Acceptance, Understanding and Integration (CTAAUI). The TAAUI and CTAAUI are simple and practical tools to resolve any severe physical or mental disorder if unconscious resistance is handled correctly. These tools help the old brain find and process the information independently and include using the rational brain to integrate it back by giving birth to further knowledge and new neural connections, resulting in inner peace and harmony.

Thus, this reinforces the purpose to live "now and here" and at the same time accepting and integrating the client's life history. In other words, it is the satisfaction, acceptance and integration of the past experiences and lessons without guilt or shame and, at the same time, acceptance, and recognition of living his whole life as the only pathway to reach his present age. It helps the client understand the importance of being in the driver's seat of his life by removing the mas of victimhood. All past decisions are accepted and appreciated without guilt or remorse. He stops living as though he were given a life sentence of repentance: "I could have, would have, should have". He experiences deep down in his heart his life story from birth to this present moment as the only pathway (and not other) to arrive at this point of his life. He accepts, experiences, and learns, and he then takes the reins of his life back into his hands to fully control his life the way he desires. It is also the unconscious acceptance and integration of the past solutions/experiences as worthy and not as anxiety or unhealthy behaviours or attitudes. He can find and change his solutions according to his present-day needs. It is a reconfirmation of "Self" with lots of choices.

Every disease is a process, and every therapy is a process. Likewise, every patient is a world, and every therapy is a world.

Every patient looks forward to understanding the world he created a long time ago and its corresponding present-day consequences. He cannot remember the moments he constructed the roots, nor can he access them as they have become part of long-term memory. Most of the time, he created that world during early ages to protect himself or perhaps because he felt lonely. (Be advised, at that time, he did not have the mature analytical awareness of an adult to understand the difference among right and wrong, positive and negative, or correct and incorrect. Later in life, through a therapeutic process, he can access and analyze the reasons to create and integrate them).

They become the regular controller of everyday life, affecting, and influencing ideas, thoughts, decisions, and actions, limiting their freedom or free will. It further creates anxiety, depression, or something similar and opens the pathway to mental or physical deterioration. He does not understand the origin of his mental or physical disorder. His need to get rid of the symptoms as quickly as possible accelerates because he wants to live a peaceful and calm life that is socially accepted by everyone around him.

Since every therapy is a world, a therapeutic process also creates a world with its own unique structure, research, and tools to handle the patient's world. Those two worlds can compete, or they can work together. They can use the process to relieve the symptoms of disease and finish the therapeutic process commonly known as goals of therapy, or they can open the possibility to understand and reverse the process of the disease and its origin while accessing early childhood or intrauterine memories which contain the seed of the mental or physical illness. The latter approach has helped more in finding permanent solutions than the previous one.

Every therapist plays a vital role in handling a patient's disorder. The success or failure of creating a therapeutic world around a patient's world entirely depends upon therapist's training, available therapeutic tools, experience, authenticity, safe and effective use of self (SEUS) and the correct handling of situations leading to transference or counter-transference. The integration must be done without guilt, punishment, or forgiveness. It is key to restoring and incorporating past unexpressed and unrecognized parts of self through Analysis, Acceptance, Absolution (reconciliation) and Application.

The therapist must accept the client unconditionally without any moral, legal, or visual evaluation of symptoms, age, sex, or appearance. He needs to have the scientific approach and appropriate in-depth knowledge of the applied therapeutic models and methods.

The therapist and his message must be positive and positively tuned (authentic). It has highest consideration in therapy because it transcends the therapist's attitude and unconscious beliefs.

The therapist must have the perception of self and the patient, working now and here (time and space) without prejudice and with all 18 senses opened.

The therapist should believe in miracles. He must think openly about the patient's still prodigious possibilities to make unexpected changes because each prognosis and expectation can be part of a transference and countertransference system. They can create a self-fulfilling prophecy effect, causing the patient to employ the same perspective as what the therapist has in mind about the patient.

An excellent therapeutic process always tries to create a balance between two hemispheres, instead of conscious or unconscious struggles and conflicts. Every experience (no matter positive or negative) and the expression of that experience through different emotions in life is essential. Past is important, the present is important, and the future is also important. The unconscious mind has a circular memory, and it is constantly creating thoughts and making decisions based on first life experiences. They just cannot be ignored or suppressed with rationalization. An excellent therapeutic process connects with all parts of the brain. It works together to accept, analyze, absolve, apply, and integrate all available memories, emotions, thoughts, or experiences be they considered negative or positive.

I invite you to read these two great case studies. I used Integrative Therapy of In-Depth Psychology by Dr. Werner Meinhold on both cases. The first mental health case is about a person who felt strong rejection and disgust throughout his life towards his mother. Even after going through many different therapeutic methods, he still could not feel his mother's love and continued feeling ups and downs of anxiety and depression.

The second case started with a mental health issue but ended with the disintegration of a tumour. This case study shows how mental health issues can heal physical illnesses too. This case study is also published in detail in my Amazon International Best Seller, "The Unseen Wisdom of the Unborn."

I have changed my clients' names to protect their privacy, and they have given me their consent to publish their therapeutic journey with the pleasure of helping others.

How Peter discovered his mother's love?

Peter came to me and described how difficult it has been for him to love his mother. He said that although his mother has always tried to do the best for him, he feels that she does not love him, and consequently, he suffers anxiety, depression, and rejection.

He confessed that he has been to many therapists who have helped him discover the connection between his mother and his dissatisfaction and struggle with his romantic relationships, but that awareness is not enough.

He further described he has learnt to manage his anxiety and depression with coping techniques to fill in everyday activities but feels an emptiness in whatever he does. He is going through sentiments of unworthiness, low self-esteem and sometimes thoughts relating to self-harm.

We discussed the different therapeutic possibilities. Peter happily accepted that he needed to experience something new, which will help him make unconscious conscious and discover the seeds of his present-day symptoms.

The first few sessions helped him open shut off memories and awareness of hidden patterns working underneath and controlling his life. The connections related to anxiety, depression and other symptoms and their relationship to early childhood conditioning and relationship with mother ended up in lots of "aha moments." He was amazed at how his anxiety and other symptoms starting to diminish, and suddenly he started feeling more mental stability and peace. However, he had some worst outbursts before reaching that state of inner calmness. It is natural to experience the ups and downs of symptoms when we work with seeds of the problem, and I explained to him before starting the therapy. Making unconscious conscious helped him get along better with his present girlfriend, and he started creating more openness and understanding towards his mother.

Suddenly, his subconscious mind opened the memories connected to his mother's relationship during a session. It was time to access maybe, the most crucial part of his therapeutic journey till so far after all those years. It is when a plane starts a landing process, and the passenger feels the turbulence.

He recalls the memory connected to 3 months of his chronological age where his mother is breast-feeding him. Still, she is not looking at him; instead, she is busy talking to his siblings, and he feels rejection and sadness because he is not the priority for his mother, and his siblings are more important than him in the eyes of his mother. At the same time, he started laughing while reliving those memories because as an adult, he is now able to rationally analyze the situation which he could not do when he was three months old.

After finishing the session, he shared his feelings. "Atul, I have mixed sentiments of anger and laughter. It is like I am divided into two parts. My other part, who I would call a little Peter, is mad at his mother, and my adult part is laughing at this situation. I have a desire to fight with my mother; why she did that to me? At the same time, I am laughing this small, wrongly interpreted experience by my little self that has caused years of anger, pain, and anxiety. I am shocked, and I never thought that this could be one of the biggest causes of not loving my mother."

He also asked if this could also be why he feels a rivalry with his siblings. I politely replied that this is his quest, and he must find his answers and is already on the pathway to get them and needs to be a little more patient. We both agreed that it would take some time to process and settle down, and that is why our session is not twenty minutes or an hour session, but it is a weekly session or a session of 167 hours.

That week he had lots of ups and downs, and he called me a few times that his anxiety levels have gone up, and he feels like throwing up many times. I explained that it is a natural part of the process because living with these symptoms has become his comfort zone. It is also an unconscious pathological way of connecting with his mother. At the same time, he is expressing what he has not been able to define for years, and that is why a good therapist accepts unconditionally every patient with his symptoms because he is complete with his symptoms. They are the pathways to the seeds and healing.

A few more sessions helped him to understand and to move into a state of inner peace. At the same time, his relationship with his siblings and parents, especially the mother, took on a new understanding and connection. He started taking more interest in his everyday life events. His confidence and self-worth had a dramatic boost, and his work performance also got better.

I can never forget that session when finally, he deciphered the unconscious's depths and resolved his relationship issues with his mother. Please note that there had been other situations between three months old and his present age that contributed to the present-day symptoms and to his stormy relationship with his mother. We worked on all those events individually to close that final chapter with the mother.

I remember he was a bit nervous that day before the session, and I could predict that something would pop up that he has not experienced before. We started the session, and we went back to the same age but this time, he had more confidence and peace than before. This time, he did not want to fight with his mother, nor did he feel bad, but rather he tried to understand what stopped him from loving his mother. It became possible by making visible what has been invisible in the story of his life.

He went back to that time when he was three months old, and this time his subconscious mind gave access to the hidden psychic level by remembering what Mom was saying to the kids. He now, with his adult mind, can rationalize it and integrate it with absolution.

He started crying and shared, "I did not know that my mother loved me so much. She is telling my siblings to go and play somewhere else because they are making noise, and she is not able to feed me, and I need her attention."

Nothing else was required as he discovered a deep, loving, and natural bond with his mother, and now there is no need to write further about how this experience changed his life. Interesting, isn't it?

Now you can experience how problems are created on an unconscious level and at the same time how all the solutions are also hiding inside us on an unconscious level. Would it not be great to tap into it? I can write a whole encyclopedia on this topic but still it will not be enough.

I decided to share this case study from my book The Unseen Wisdom of the Unborn described from pages 105 to 109. Although I shared the details from the actual therapeutic sessions as described by my client, here I provide an abridged version of what caused the tumour at the end of the client's testimonial. I witnessed a wonder when I observed how malignant energies could create a tumour.

The whole-life therapeutic process surfaced new ideas, new surprises, and new experiences that culminated into an amazing event. She shared her experiences related to disintegrating a tumour in her body. I have her enthusiastic and express permission to share her incredible story with you.

It is incredible to me to realize that the conditions experienced in a mother's womb could also act as fertile grounds for a benign tumour to take root and grow later in her life. I will call my client Alba to respect her privacy and to protect her real identity.

In April 2006, Alba started yoga classes with me. She revealed that she suffered from pain in her right knee. After a few classes, we discussed and explored the symbolism related to her knee pain, and she recognized the connection and agreed to begin the whole life therapy process under conscious hypnosis based on Dr. Werner Meinhold's techniques and guidelines. The therapeutic process ended in April 2010 with around 200 sessions.

She had been under the care of a psychiatrist who had been treating her for the past six months for depression and anxiety. She was hospitalized for five days to undergo sleep therapy, received weekly sessions, and took many medications for months thereafter without any improvement in her symptoms. She said, "I carried out only what the doctor told me to do because I wanted to be released from the hospital. The anxieties continued, I felt sadness inside me, I did not find any peace; moreover, I could not find any solutions to what led me into this state." She also disclosed her difficult relationship with her parents and siblings.

Approximately 15 years ago, she began to experience irregular menstrual periods. Later, blood tests results detected higher prolactin levels and she was diagnosed with Polycystic Ovary Syndrome. Her gynecologist prescribed medications to be taken daily for the rest of her life. Eventually, a small tumour on Sella Turcica in the Pituitary gland was discovered. The most astounding part was that we always talked about her fears, resentments, anxieties, fantasies, and realities, but never openly discussed the benign tumour she had. Nor did I have much experience in this area and thought of it as more as being the domain of a medical professional or a neurosurgeon. For me, psychotherapy was a treatment for those who suffer from mental health problems. While in therapy with me, my client faithfully took her medication to menstruate and to manage high prolactin levels, until her doctor asked her to stop it completely.

During our second year of therapy the tumour grew a little bit more. Gradually, over time, she began to make room for peace in her life. Here is her story, in her words:

"During these fantastic, very often, difficult and emotionally strong moments – I learned to know myself better, to accept me as I am and to love myself. I learned to look at and accept my parents and siblings as they are: human beings with successes and mistakes; I learned to look at them with love, try not to judge them but to understand them, I learned to forgive what had to be forgiven and accept what I had lived and to understand what I lived it for. It was learning at every moment, in every circumstance. During therapy, and after finishing it, I have been able to move closer to my father with love, respect, and acceptance, and no longer with anger and resentment which I had felt towards him, because during the therapy, I understood many things related to his attitude towards me, and it opened my heart. I could also accept the alienation of my brother and accept it as it is, to forgive him for not wanting to get closer to me; I understood, and I stopped feeling the pain of rejection. Likewise, with my mom, I could heal some resentment that I had kept very deep inside me. I started talking and moving closer to my sister with whom I had a strong conflict and we had not talked for a long time."

She continues, "In therapy, I realized why I had to maintain stormy loving relationships. I used to harm myself by getting involved with the wrong people who hurt me and above all,

I allowed them to hurt me. Based on that understanding, I was able to get away from my best friend because his friendship was not convenient, and I got the courage to say enough and think first of my own well-being, and from then onwards, I am in peace, and now I am not looking for someone to hurt me, because now I know that I only deserve to receive love and I can give love. As therapy advanced, I knew a little more of myself, I was learning to value more, to love, to understand people close to me, and how my whole environment, my beliefs and my way of seeing and living life had influenced me to be who I was at that time."

"It is incredible to look back now on how I was a conflicted person, sometimes sad and depressed, dependent on others to take decisions, looking for others' approval, fearful to make certain decisions. Right after the therapy, I realized that I am the one who chooses which path to follow. Previously, I chose the difficult path, with sadness and despair, with suicide attempts, and with frustrations. The path which I now travel and enjoy is full of happiness, optimism, internalizing every day, living, and breathing life with the open heart, with the healthy body, with an open mind and looking for new options, with more freedom of heart to love and letting others love me too. Part of that beautiful process of self-awareness led me to realize that when I was twelve years old, I was very afraid of growing up, moving from girl to become a woman, for different experiences and situations that I would discover and understand as the therapy sessions advanced.

All of this led me to understand that it was that fear that made me generate prolactin problems and consequently appearance of the tumour in the pituitary gland. This great understanding led me to the healing process, I understood and accepted my fears, embraced them, forgave myself and moved ahead, and to the surprise of my attending physician, the tumour disappeared, my prolactin stabilized, and I stopped taking medication."

"I remember the time after the exam, my doctor saw the results and was surprised. He said that for him there was no other reason than a miracle because it was one in a million chance for the tumour to disappear and for everything to become normalized in such a short time. He could not accept that working on my self-awareness helped me to heal, but he told me that he is not completely ruling out that possibility. From that time the test results were positive until now, ten years have passed, and my body works very well, I have regular periods without the use of medicines."

I share this testimonial with you because I think it is a call to awaken our consciousness. We need to realize that thoughts and emotions manifest in our body, and that when we know ourselves, we help ourselves to heal, to care, to love, to recognize that we are holistic beings (body, mind, and spirit). The most beautiful part of this was the experiences lived by my client during her intrauterine life. She discovered moments of premature delivery as well as bitterness of rejection due to being an unwanted baby, all of which formed the future basis of a tumour within her. During her intrauterine life she felt rejected by her mother and decided to take birth during her 7th month in the womb. She vividly remembers her mother conversing with the doctor about the fact that the baby should be born after 9 months; otherwise, she might be born with some part of her body missing, causing her to be further rejected by her siblings and parents. Now she wants to go back but can't. With overwhelming frustration that she is not complete, she hits her forehead against a bone, which hurt her a lot. Although she was born prematurely, she had all body parts intact; but later in life that forehead incident transformed into a benign tumour in the same spot where she had hit her head during the birthing process. Under what circumstances could it have become malignant?

The integrative therapy of depth psychology as developed by Dr. Werner Meinhold, has also helped me to explore the depths of unconscious and find new answers to understand the basic need for a disease. As a therapist, I have used these tools during the therapeutic process to help thousands of my clients deal with their mental and physical issues. One of my best experiences has been to go through the whole life therapy process which helped me to access deepest parts of human consciousness in intrauterine life which further helped me not only to resolve many present-day issues but also resulted in experiencing reconfirmation of self with many options. Since then, the results have been amazing working with different clients regardless of their health condition. After exploring the depths of their own unconscious mind, my clients have been empowered to opt to discontinue the disease and break up those malignant connections that created it in the first place.

Here is the list of diseases which can be treated with Integrative Therapy of in-depth psychology.

1) Addictions: Adiposity, alcoholism, drugs, drugs and nicotine, television, electronic games, etc.
2) Allergies.
3) Increased performance on mental and physical area, such as memory, concentration, sports.
4) Bulimia
5) Cancer (as a measure of support and healing)
6) Functional heart problems
7) Concentration problems
8) Sleeping problems
9) Psychological issues, e.g., depression
10) Sexual problems

11) Auto-immune diseases, such as ulcerative colitis, Rheumatism, multiple sclerosis etc.
12) Skin diseases
13) Stomach and intestine ailments especially ulcer, constipation etc.
14) Diseases of the senses
14) Motor system diseases, such as carpal tunnel syndrome, tics etc.
15) State of pain
16) Bedwetting
17) Repeated infections
18) Paralysis and to support rehabilitation, for example after a stroke or an accident
19) Fears: Mortal anguish, embarrassment, fear of contact, public nervousness, agoraphobia, fear of exams, fear of public speaking, etc.
20) Migraines and other functional headaches
21) Neurosis
22) Obsessions
23) Burns.
24) Stuttering.

Sometimes THIPP can be applied on other diseases when advisable, for example, when there are drug allergies or resistance, or because other means have failed. With all these broad fields of application, one must not forget that this therapy does not have the "goal to fight against disease" hiding the symptoms.

I hope this last chapter helped you to understand how miracles can occur if we work together with our mind and body and consciousness. If modern scientific studies can be persuaded to be more open to spending some money on researching therapeutic methods to help understand and treat the person as a whole, then it would be a giant step in the right direction. For the first time in human history, we would be able to unite science, politico-economics, and healthcare to achieve a common goal that would lead to the bringing peace and wholeness to individuals and improve the overall state of our nation as well.

"I have concluded that I need to love and accept myself first."

Atul Mehra

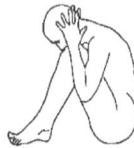

Conclusion

I feel thrilled and satisfied to share all this information with you; together, we have taken a step forward, and I am sure many of you now have a profound glimpse of the human body and the games played by our psyche between health and disease to maintain the body survival.

Many of you must have experienced some personal connection to the information shared in this book and in your own lived experiences. Now that we have arrived at this book's end, the origin of disease and healing is no longer a mystery. It should no longer be a thing for you to get scared of but a pathway to inner growth. The purpose of life is to take awareness of yourself, understand yourself from different angles, merge good and bad life events as experiences, and then use the lessons learned in everyday life.

When you reject yourself physically, mentally, or spiritually, you divide yourself, and inner conflict appears. If there is no early solution, it can lead to struggle, and struggle leads to anger, anger leads to aggression, aggression leads to violence, violence leads to hurt and hurt brings pain and suffering, and those cause mental ailments such as anxiety, depression and that further translates into physical illnesses. The origin of happiness is inside you because you are the most important person in the universe. Everything exists because you exist; without you, the space you occupy would be empty. The idea of living a happy and healthy life is first to start taking care of yourself. Love and accept yourself. Live a positive life and at the same time understand and learn the methods or techniques to integrate negative because then only you can become one, whole and complete within you. You become In-dependent and not out-dependent.

The origin of human consciousness at the beginning passes through experiences of love without judgement. The love brings you into existence, and when the love is expressed badly or finds an incorrect way to express itself, then it changes into a something opposite and creates experiences related to pain and suffering. The definitions of health and disease become parallel to each other, and the unconscious mind tries to communicate through a whatever means. The external factors such as society, culture and religion create conditions to get accepted and the "normal" of life control and discover conscious or unconscious ways to resist self-love. Self-love and acceptance collaborate themselves through unconscious hooks and find ugly ways to survive while making noise that your past experiences are holding you back and they are not letting you enjoy your life to the fullest because you are carrying the heavy burdens of the past still on your shoulders. The more you try to avoid or get rid of it, stronger they become. They transform themselves into mental, physical, or spiritual symptoms and then it is when the need for disease arises because every disease is an unspoken and unrecognized part of the self.

That is when the process of recognizing the self starts because if you create your disease, you can heal it too.

Everything is inside you, all your questions and all your answers. You start understanding how you have ignored yourself and given others priority in your life and sacrificed so much by looking for validation and acceptance from others. The fear of rejection made you do things that you would not have done otherwise. You did not speak for yourself, and it was almost impossible for you to say no. You lived your life till now conditionally, first to have and then to be. Now it is time for you to stand up, start taking care of yourself and make peace with each one in your heart, including your parents, with reconfirmation of self and many options. The solutions you found in the past to express yourself now are no longer valid because you grew up biologically, and mentally you got frozen in the past. That frozen part controls the most important decisions of your everyday life. It is time to take the stand, and it is time to take control of your life Now and Here. As the story goes, the little ugly and weak duckling grows and converts into a beautiful and intelligent swan.

Some information for you to consider: -

1. The person creates the disease so he can heal it too.
2. There is no need to be afraid of the disease but accept it and find pathways to learn the lesson so you can say goodbye to it.
3. The disease is an expression of the Unconscious Self. It is a small little child frozen in time who, during the earliest moments of his life, felt rejected and unwanted according to his limited or no rational interpretation of those moments.
4. The anxieties, depression or other physical or mental symptoms are expressions of rejected part or parts of self because you create your disease. You cannot buy it on a credit card, for cash or even a postdated cheque.

It is essential to find a correct therapeutic process to uncover present-day comfort zone masks by making unconscious conscious and accessing the seeds of the disease in the mother's womb. The adult analyzes those memories by processing and understanding the opposite point of view and carrying the researched information to those early childhood memories to complete the lived experience. It helps to make the invisible visible with non-local or telepathic communication while simultaneously coming out of unconscious hooks while dealing efficiently with unconscious resistance. For example, if the error is on page two, you cannot correct it on page 30.

The therapeutic process requires analysis, acceptance, absolution (reconciliation without forgiveness) and implementation of the process information in life while making peace in the heart with himself, and everyone around, including the parents, according to his belief system.

He starts living his birthright- a harmonious and peaceful life. The frozen child feels accepted and loved. He grows into a young, intelligent, balanced adult and feels connected to himself and everyone around him. His finances, relationships, career, and mental, physical, and spiritual health harmonize. During this process, all the physical and mental disturbances or discomforts can return to their original state of health, and the person can live a complete and satisfactory life in all areas of his life.

You are in the driver's seat of your life's car, and only you know how to start, drive, stop, park, and handle the steering wheel. How do you feel when someone else drives your vehicle?

Now you have all the tools, go out there in life's adventures and use them.

And finally, I would like to thank you from the bottom of my heart for joining me on this journey. I would be grateful if you want to contact me and share your ideas and questions, or even sending a note about the book would be appreciated. You can contact me through my email atul@atulmehra.com or visit my website at www.atulmehra.com.

Love and Hugs,

Atul Mehra

Author, Speaker and Psychotherapist

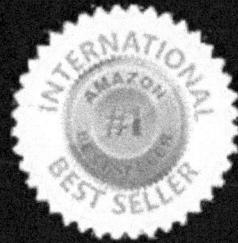

"Atul's book is a must read for every prospective parent."
- Deepak Chopra

THE UNSEEN WISDOM OF THE UNBORN

Is your future decided before birth?

INTERNATIONAL
AMAZON
#1
BEST SELLER

Atul K. Mehra

Second Edition

www.ingramcontent.com/pod-product-compliance
Lightning Source LLC
Chambersburg PA
CBHW071233020426
42333CB00015B/1456